Halperin/Graser/Rogoff/Plekavich

Mastering the Art of Complete Dentures

Mastering the Art of Complete Dentures

Alexander R. Halperin, D.D.S.
Lecturer in Prosthetic Dentistry;
formerly, Assistant Professor of Prosthetic Dentistry,
Harvard School of Dental Medicine, Boston, Massachusetts;
formerly, Assistant Professor of Prosthodontics, The University of Texas Health
Science Center at San Antonio, Dental School, San Antonio, Texas

Gerald N. Graser, D.D.S., M.S., F.A.C.D.
Chairman, Department of Prosthodontics, Eastman Dental Center, Rochester, New York;
Associate Professor of Clinical Dentistry and Dental Research, University of
Rochester School of Medicine and Dentistry, Rochester, New York

Gary S. Rogoff, D.D.S., M.S.
Assistant Clinical Professor, Department of Implant Research,
Forsyth Dental Center, Boston, Massachusetts;
Clinical Instructor in Prosthetic Dentistry,
Harvard School of Dental Medicine, Boston, Massachusetts;
formerly, Assistant Research Professor of Complete Denture Prosthetics,
Tufts University School of Dental Medicine, Boston, Massachusetts

Edward J. Plekavich, D.D.S., M.S.
Associate Professor, Department of Fixed Prosthodontics,
Georgetown University School of Dentistry, Washington, D.C.

quintessence books

Quintessence Publishing Co., Inc. 1988
Chicago, Berlin, London, São Paulo, Hong Kong, and Tokyo

Illustrations are the artist's representations. Exact accuracy has sometimes been sacrificed to better explain a concept.

Library of Congress Cataloging-in-Publication Data

Mastering the art of complete dentures.

Includes bibliographies and index.
1. Complete dentures. I. Halperin, Alexander R.
[DNLM: 1. Denture, Complete. 2. Mouth, Edentulous—rehabilitation. WU 530 M423]
RK656.M385 1988 617.6'92 87-29237
ISBN 0-86715-185-4

quintessence books

Senior photographic consultant: Harvey Segall, Wrentham, MA
Copy editor: Sue R. Bricker, Sharon, MA
Dental laboratory technician: Regis Andrews, C.D.T., Nashua, NH
Clinical photographer: Steven N. Cohen, D.M.D., Canton, MA
Graphic artist: Mary Beth Antin, Needham, MA

Lithography: Toppan Printing Co. (S) Pte. Ltd., Jurong, Singapore
Composition: Graphic World, Inc., St. Louis, MO
Printing and binding: BookCrafters, Chelsea, MI
Printed in the U. S. A.

Contents

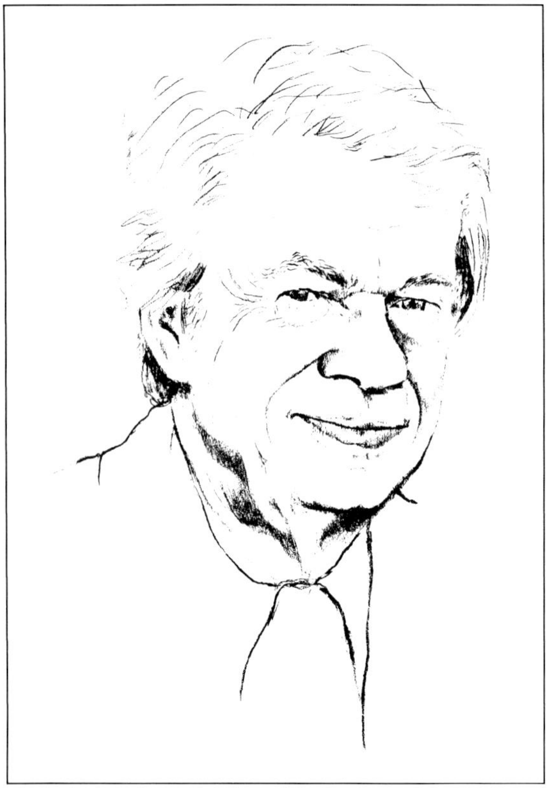

1911–1987

Dedicated to the memory of Allen A. Brewer, whose contributions to dentistry far transcend the teaching of prosthodontics. He provided an education in life as well as dentistry for those who were fortunate enough to have studied with him.

Foreword

The late Allen Brewer personified many of the characteristics of prosthodontic excellence. He was a superb clinician and a dedicated teacher, and countless dentists in North America and Europe benefited from his enormous clinical acumen. His recent passing might have impoverished dental education had not a cadre of his old students undertaken the task of synthesizing so much of Dr. Brewer's clinical teaching and experience. This book is the result, and it is a real pleasure to have it as such a tidy and potent reinforcement of the art of making complete dentures. It is also a very good read. It is clear, concise, and lucid. Above all it deals with the topic in a realistic and practical manner. It balances analysis with step-by-step "how to" sections, clear diagrams with particularly relevant illustrations. The chapters are spiced with the pearls of clinical wisdom which Allen Brewer was so famous for.

The four authors are capable and experienced educators and prosthodontists in their own right. Like their teacher, they too have already enriched prosthodontic education. Their initiative in writing this book is therefore commendable, and our discipline is much the better for it.

George A. Zarb, B.Ch.D., D.D.S., M.S., M.S., F.R.C.D.(C)
Professor and Head of Prosthodontics
Faculty of Dentistry
University of Toronto

Preface

After several years of practice most dentists realize that prosthodontics is more than a simple "take an impression and send it to the lab" procedure. If we want to ensure that patient satisfaction and making removable prosthodontics are the rewarding parts of our practice that they should be, we have to follow an approach that will give us *predictable* results. That is the thrust of this book.

This is not a book about making complete dentures faster or less costly, but a book about making good dentures with better techniques. The book contains a unique set of empirically derived artistic principles combined with scientifically verifiable facts. It is a distinctive blend of art and science.

The authors of *Mastering the Art of Complete Dentures* were fortunate enough to have learned firsthand about prosthodontics from Dr. Allen Brewer. He was a Diplomate of the American Board of Prosthodontics and an active, contributing member of many prosthodontic organizations. He served in the United States Air Force from 1949 to 1965, after several years in private practice in Illinois. Toward the end of his career in the Air Force, he was head of the Department of Prosthodontics in the USAF School of Aerospace Medicine. The research he conducted there, along with the related publications he produced, led to the growth of his international reputation in his profession. It was at this time that he began developing his precision techniques for making complete dentures. In 1966 and 1967, he was Chief of the Central Dental Laboratory at the Veterans Administration in Washington, D.C. He then retired from government service and founded the Department of Prosthodontics at the Eastman Dental Center in Rochester, New York, where he held the position of Chairman until 1977. It was at Eastman that the authors were his students.

Dr. Brewer was the coauthor of *Overdentures*, published in 1975, and authored several articles in *The Journal of Prosthetic Dentistry*. During his years in the Air Force and at Eastman, he was involved in research in all areas of prosthodontics, with several publications to his credit. His many contributions were formally recognized in 1968, when he was given the Jerome Schweitzer Research Award for Excellence in Research in Prosthodontics.

Although formally retired, Dr. Brewer maintained an active interest in prosthodontics and continued to teach at Eastman Dental Center until his death in 1987.

The authors have had the experience of utilizing Dr. Brewer's precision techniques on thousands of denture patients. Each author has taught both dental students and postgraduate prosthodontic residents. Much of the material presented in this book has been effectively used as teaching aids and in lecture series.

Dr. Brewer maintained that there are two ways to complete a denture: *(1)* before it is inserted, or *(2)* after it is inserted. The techniques in this book describe the completion of dentures *before* insertion. Predictability of results can be achieved only in this manner, by concentrating efforts in the right place at each step during the treatment, and by not saving procedures for the postinsertion adjustment period.

This book is organized by the sequence of procedures that should be followed to construct complete dentures. Chapter 1 describes a systematic method of patient examination, diagnosis, and prognosis. Chapters 2 through 6 describe and illustrate impressioning procedures. These procedures use a selective tissue placement technique by which the dentist can determine which denture-bearing tissues receive selected amounts of tissue placement.

The rationale and technique for using completed denture bases in accomplishing all jaw relation records and subsequent fabrication procedures is explained in chapter 7. The accuracy of the centric jaw relation record is directly related to the stability, retention, and fit of the record bases upon which it is made.

In chapter 8, a sophisticated and precise technique for verifying the accuracy of the centric jaw relation records using Centric Check Points is described.

Chapters 9 through 12 discuss the importance of tooth selection and arrangement and introduce laboratory procedures for the techniques in this book.

The denture-insertion appointment is discussed in chapter 13.

This book will complement existing prosthodontic textbooks. Each chapter presents highly refined, step-by-step procedures for impression making, defining maxillomandibular relationships, and tooth selection and arrangement. Supportive material on removable partial dentures is in chapter 14.

Dr. Allen Brewer's philosophy and techniques are described in these chapters with, we hope, the spirit and energy with which he himself studied and taught. Dentists and laboratory technicians who read this book will be able to take advantage of his knowledge and experience in accomplishing dental procedures with expertise.

Acknowledgments

We would like to thank all of the people who directly and indirectly were involved in helping us bring this book to fruition. Harvey Segall, with his exceptional professional skills, designed special photographic setups, directed and advised us, developed our film, and printed all the photographs.

A special thank you goes to Sue Bricker, who put her valuable writing and editing experience and talent to work for us. She edited, rewrote, and organized our work, developing a manuscript suitable to send to our publisher.

We'd also like to thank Dr. Gail Halperin for her invaluable editing, advice, and critique of the manuscript.

Regis Andrews, one of the most meticulous and talented dental technicians we have met, provided assistance with our laboratory procedures, offered the laboratory technician's point of view, and participated in many marathon photographic sessions.

Dr. Steven Cohen assisted us with our clinical photography, and Mary Beth Antin, a talented graphic artist, provided all the illustrations for the book.

Additionally, we would like to acknowledge the time and efforts of Elaine Silberman, our demonstration patient, and Richard C. Manor, M.A., C.D.T., who assisted with some of our laboratory procedures.

The encouragement and tolerance of our wives, Dr. Gail Halperin, Nancy Graser, Sue Bricker, and Cordelia Plekavich, cannot be overemphasized. Throughout the various stages of the book's development, their thoughts and support allowed us to put into reality what may only have lived on as a dream.

And a special thanks to our children—Laurie and Karen Halperin; Geoffrey, John, Joanna, and Suzanne Graser; Melissa Bricker-Rogoff; and Dina Plekavich—for tolerating our inattentiveness.

Chapter 1

Examination, Diagnosis, and Prognosis

The time to determine how successfully complete dentures can be made for a patient is before treatment and before fabrication of the dentures. That is also the time to inform the patient of the prognosis—of how well he will be able to wear the dentures and of what kinds of problems he might expect to encounter. Only then can the patient decide whether he wants new dentures made. Some patients may be willing to accept less than ideal results if properly prepared for the outcome.

Because of the importance of presenting an accurate prognosis before beginning treatment, an adequate examination must be completed and a correct diagnosis must be made. It is the dentist's responsibility to then inform his patient of these findings prior to fabricating the dentures. In the medical profession, for example, if a patient requires coronary bypass surgery, he has the right to ask the surgeon the following questions: "How successful do you think the surgery will be?" and "What kind of life will I have after the operation?" (Fig. 1-1). The cardiac surgeon will then accurately inform the patient and/or his family of the outcome, thus enabling the patient and his family to decide whether or not to proceed with the surgery.

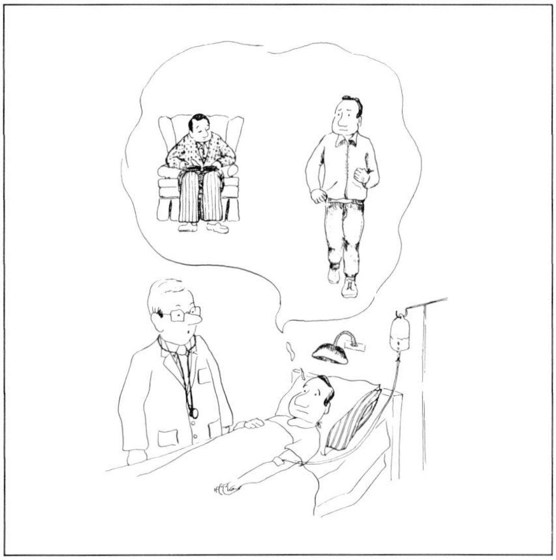

Fig. 1-1 Understanding the prognosis for a coronary bypass operation will help the patient make the decision of whether or not to have surgery. Likewise, a dentist should be able to inform patients of their prognosis for wearing complete dentures prior to beginning treatment.

Likewise, the dentist should be able to inform a patient of his prognosis for wearing complete dentures. This information may influence the patient's decisions about whether or not to have new dentures made, or may prepare the patient for a less than ideal treatment result.

In making a prognosis it is our job to determine each patient's expectations and needs. One patient may require that special attention be given to the appearance of the dentures, while another patient may only be concerned that he can eat well. We should gauge the purposes for which an individual wants to use his teeth, and we should then tell the patient whether or not he will be able to use his dentures for those purposes.

The population of denture-wearing patients can be roughly divided into three groups based upon the difficulty of treatment:

Group 1: relatively easy. For about 70% of all denture patients, the dentist can make some significant compromises and still be successful with the treatment. For example, denture bases may be over- or underextended, or esthetics and phonetics can be less than ideal, and yet those patients may be happy and wear such dentures without complaint.

Group 2: somewhat difficult. About 20% of the denture-wearing population are not as easy to treat and satisfy. They have some difficulty wearing dentures. If one or more of the essential aspects of treatment is overlooked or done incorrectly for the patient's needs, the chance for success is lessened and the patient will continue to have problems. The task is, first, to identify the particular problems, and second, to determine what, if anything, can be done to remedy them.

Group 3: difficult. The remaining 10% have behavioral (psychological) and/or anatomic factors that make patient satisfaction difficult or impossible to achieve. This means that this group will be more demanding and difficult to treat to its satisfaction. It is often these patients who come for their first visit carrying multiple dentures made by several dentists. For these people, the loss of their own natural teeth is one of the worst tragedies of their lives.[1]

Prognosis rating scale

Within this chapter patient examination and evaluation are divided into four sections: gross appraisal of the patient; patient needs and expectations; medical, psychological, and behavioral considerations; and anatomic and physiologic factors. Within each chapter specific criteria for judging prognoses are discussed. After looking at the criteria, say, for patient needs and expectations, it should be possible to form an overall prognosis, and it is our suggestion that a numerical rating system such as the following be applied:

1 = Most favorable prognosis
2 = Integral on scale
3 = Least favorable prognosis

Similarly, a numerical prognosis value can be assigned for each of the other three areas. By combining the scores of all four areas, you can make an overall prognosis for the patient. The separate and overall pretreatment prognostic ratings should then be entered onto the patient's chart as a permanent record.

In determining a prognosis by this scale you must understand that not all isolated factors carry equal weight. One important negative factor could outweigh the positive ones and mean certain failure for a patient. A patient may have a No. 1 rating based upon anatomy but at the same time have a No. 3 psychological prognosis. If the latter factor carries more weight, the overall prognosis would not be good. The factors analyzed in this chapter are meant to be guides to patient evaluation, not numerical hard-and-fast rules.

After treatment is completed and after the patient has worn the dentures for a significant amount of time (approximately three months), you can judge your pretreatment prognosis for that patient by considering several questions. Were you correct in predicting how successfully this patient would be able to wear dentures? If not, why not? What problem(s) did you and the patient encounter that were not expected or foreseen? By reviewing your success in forecasting the results of treatment you can better educate yourself for future patient care. The review process gives you the opportunity to step back and evaluate your examination and diagnostic procedures as well as your denture techniques.

Overall appraisal of the patient

Dress, carriage, and poise

The examination begins when you meet the patient, and with your overall physical appraisal of the patient. This is an easy, relaxed way to start your evaluation. Keep in mind that this first meeting with the patient is important and, ideally, should not take place with the patient in the dental

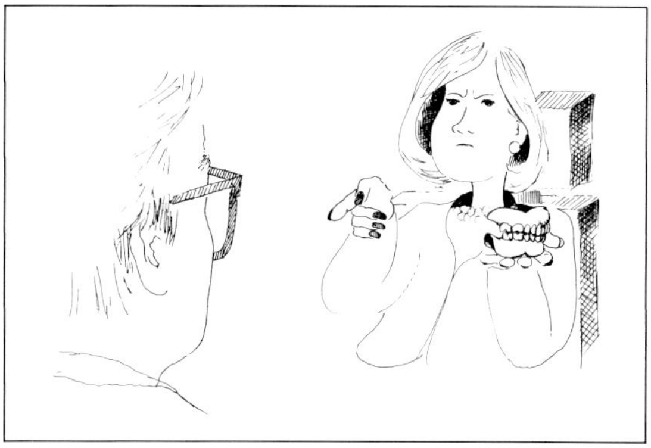

Fig. 1-2 This patient may eventually blame the dentist for all of her problems—dental and nondental. It is important to find this out before beginning treatment.

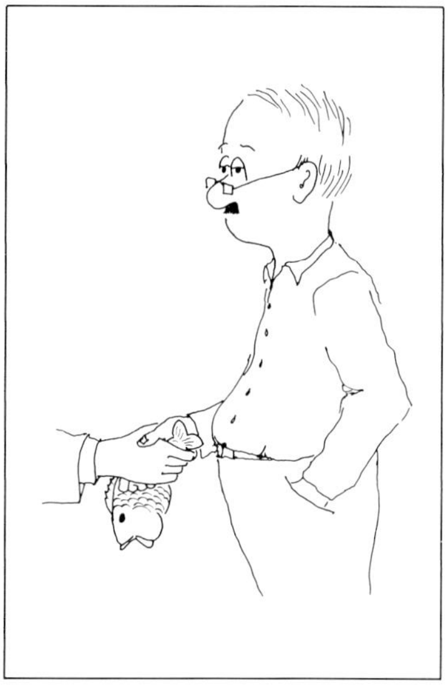

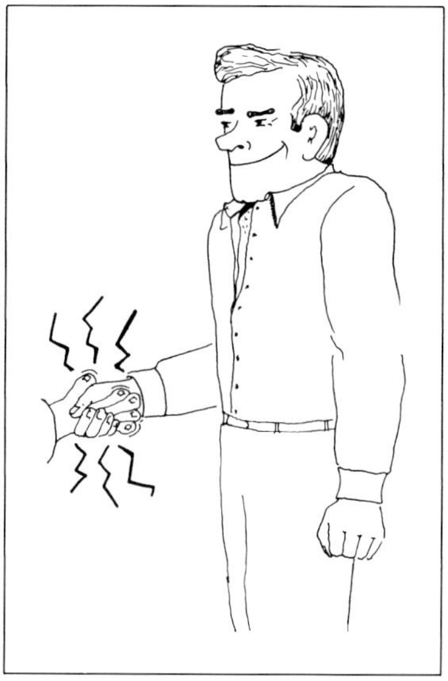

Figs. 1-3a and b The handshake may reveal much about the emotional state of the patient.

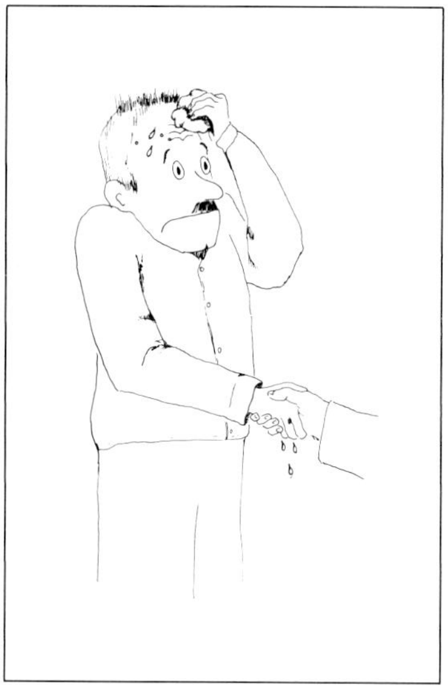

Fig. 1-3c The temperature of a patient's hand (normal or cold and clammy) can also reveal information about the patient's emotional state.

chair. Greet the patient, when possible, as he walks into a consultation room or private office.

This first place of meeting should be a pleasant environment—neat, clean, attractive, and above all, comfortable. The first meeting is private and should not be disturbed by phone calls and messages. It is very disconcerting for the patient to feel that he is competing with others for your time.

As patients walk toward us, we automatically appraise their physical characteristics—dress, carriage, poise, and apparent age. However, we might do well to keep in mind the maxim, "appearances can be deceiving." Our natural inclination might be to think, if the patient is young and attractive, that he will have the more favorable prognosis. While this may be true, it also may be possible that this patient could be more demanding. If we had to extract all of an attractive woman's remaining teeth and fabricate immediate complete dentures for her, she might later blame the denist for all of her problems, dental and nondental (Fig. 1-2).

Patients who are older or less attractive, whom we might be inclined to consider "problem" patients at first sight, may be well adjusted and busy enough with their daily activities not to be thinking constantly of themselves. Psychologically, they may be the more ideal denture patients.

There are other factors, not so obvious as appearance, to be considered when gathering information for the prognosis.

The handshake

Shaking hands with a patient may reveal much about the emotional state of the patient at the time of the dental visit. Two distinct types of handshakes are the deadfish and the viselike grip. The deadfish handshake (Fig. 1-3a) might indicate an uncooperative patient without too much interest. In contrast, the viselike grip (Fig. 1-3b) could be introducing a patient who is insecure. This patient might try impressing us with how well he could wear our dentures, or might later concentrate on trying to prove we could not do a good enough job for him. The patient offering a normal, firm handshake would probably be the easiest to get along with. Other information to be gleaned from a handshake is whether a patient's hands are hot or cold, sticky or dry. The patient with sweaty, clammy, and cold hands is likely to be anxious about the impending dental work (Fig. 1-3c).

At the same time the dentist is observing the patient's appearance, the patient is observing the dentist and the office. Although we are told in dental school to be sharp and clean, not all patients would feel comfortable with a cold and authoritative personality. We don't want to appear messy, but should make every effort to be "down-to-earth" with our patients. You and any auxiliaries who will treat the patient should use a mouthwash or breath freshener. Even when you are wearing gloves, wash your hands with a soap that leaves a pleasant scent and lack of bitter taste on the fingers. The operatory should be immaculate and uncluttered. Keep in mind that the patient examines our offices very carefully from the time he reaches the front door.

Obviously, your initial impression based upon the physical characteristics of the patient is not enough, but it may give you some insight before you gather further information, and it can help you with what you say and how you respond to the patient during your first meeting.

Aging and prognosis

Because a large percentage of patients requiring complete dentures are over the age of 60, we should carefully evaluate how the patient's age may affect his ability to wear dentures. When greeting the patient, it can be helpful to notice his apparent age as it compares to his actual age. A patient may be 72 years old but look and act as though he were 60. In this situation, the 72-year-old patient may be treated more successfully than another patient who is 60 but looks 72 and leads a rather dormant, debilitated life-style. People who are not active may tend to spend a great deal of time thinking about themselves and their problems and in consequence may be difficult to please.

The aging process can also affect the success with which a patient is able to wear complete dentures. It is not uncommon to see a 70-year-old patient who has been wearing one set of complete dentures successfully for 20 to 30 years. Although these dentures may be badly worn, unstable, and loose, the patient may not experience any discomfort or complain about either comfort or fit. Many a dentist, with confidence, proceeds to make new dentures for such a patient thinking, "How can I fail? I can certainly make something better than he is wearing." Ultimately, such an approach often does lead to failure.

Although the new dentures may be well made, the older patient simply may not adapt to them. Tissues of the older patient are significantly less resilient and elastic and have an associated loss in tissue tone. The mucosa and submucosa above the bone are thinner. This, in combination with an altered repair potential after injury, makes the tissues more susceptible to trauma with an associated delay in healing time.

Behavioral changes in the elderly compound the anatomic and histologic changes described above. As we age, there is an associated decrease in our reaction time, a slowing of our healing abilities, and a decrease in our ability to remember. Behaviorally, some elderly do not adapt well to new situations or to new prostheses such as dentures, eyeglasses, or footwear. Many aged patients want a guarantee that their new dentures will be better than what they have, but be aware that there is no guarantee.

It is also common to see daughters and sons of elderly parents seeking to please their parents by offering to have new dentures made for them (Fig. 1-4). Children may be disturbed by the parents' constant complaints about their dentures or their lack of ability to eat certain foods. They may be embarrassed by the way the dentures "clack" or by the way they look. Although the parents do complain about their dentures to their children, often they really do not want new ones made. In these situations, the dentist is making the dentures for the children's sake and not for the patient, often leading to unhappy and unsuccessful results.

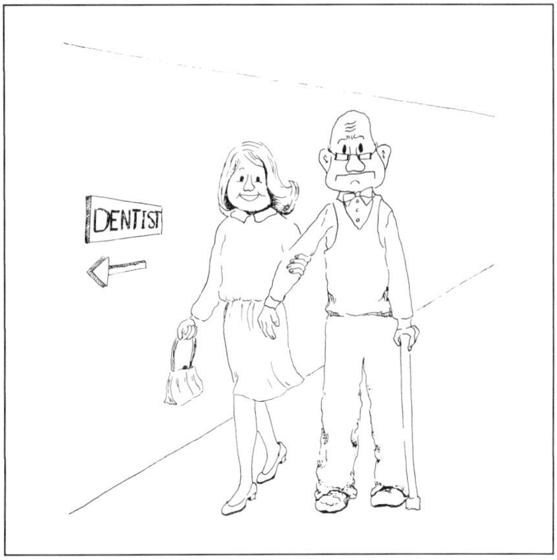

Fig. 1-4 Children of elderly parents often seek to please them by offering to have new dentures made for them. In this situation, the dentist may be making the dentures for the daughter, not her father. The prognosis in such situations is poor.

Patient needs and expectations

Questions to ask denture patients

A dental health questionnaire can be given to the patient prior to the first meeting, or it can be used as a guide for oral questions during the personal interview with the patient (Fig. 1-5). These questions allow the patient to express his reasons for seeking dental treatment. You should also ask questions pertaining to previous denture experience and personal habits. This information helps you get to know the patient prior to beginning any treatment.

Listening to the patient

A simple question such as "What can we do for you, Mrs. Smith?" or "What is the problem with your dentures?" can elicit a good deal of information. Our job is to ask the appropriate questions and then to listen (Fig. 1-6). A patient with a problem usually has no difficulty talking about it and revealing details related to the problem. Ultimately, it is our task to correlate the patient's needs and expectations with what we think we can do. Thus we arrive at the prognosis.

By listening to the patient we find out what he does for a living or hobbies and habits that he may have (Figs. 1-7a to c) . If he is a clarinet player or a singer, dentures may put him out of business or at least make it very difficult to perform with the same ease. The pipe smoker may have a problem keeping the dentures stabilized in his mouth while smoking.

Patients are likely to tell us what they expect from dentures. It is the ambition of some people to be able to eat corn on the cob or whole apples (Fig. 1-8). Although it will be possible for some patients to eat such foods, others will find it difficult or not have the ability or confidence to do it, especially when in the company of other people. Such aspirations can affect the treatment. We should be able to inform the patient whether or not he will be able to use his new dentures for this purpose.

Suggested questions to ask a new denture patient

- Why are you here for dental care?
- Who referred you to this office?
- When were your natural teeth extracted?
- Why were your teeth extracted?
- How do you feel about having lost your natural teeth?
- Did you have "immediate" dentures (was your denture placed in your mouth right after your teeth were extracted) or did you wait to have your dentures made?
- How did you manage with your first set of dentures? What problems did you have?
- Did you ever wear a partial denture? What experiences did you have with it?
- How many dentures have you had made and when?
- Do you want new dentures? Why?
- What do you *like* most about your dentures?
- What do you *dislike* most about your dentures?
- What do you expect from new dentures?
- What is the most important thing to you about wearing dentures?

  Comfort?
  Appearance?
  Chewing ability?
  The fit (how tight they are)?
  Speech?

- Is your mouth often dry, lacking saliva?
- What foods do you not eat because of your dentures?
- Do you avoid smiling or laughing? Why?
- Do you wear your dentures 24 hours a day? Why?
- Do you smoke cigarettes, pipe, or cigar?
- Do you chew gum or tobacco?
- Do you clench or brux (grind) your teeth?
- Do you play a wind instrument?
- Do you sing or act?
- Do you do public speaking?
- Do your dentures affect your occupation or hobbies? How?

Fig. 1-5 A dental health questionnaire that can be given to the patient prior to the first meeting.

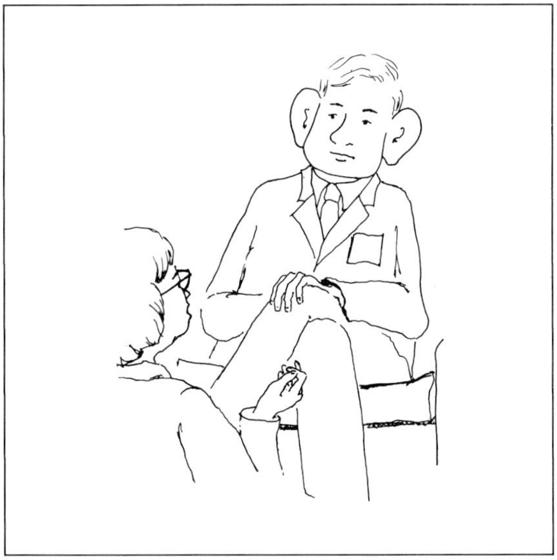

Fig. 1-6 Let the patient talk—the dentist listens.

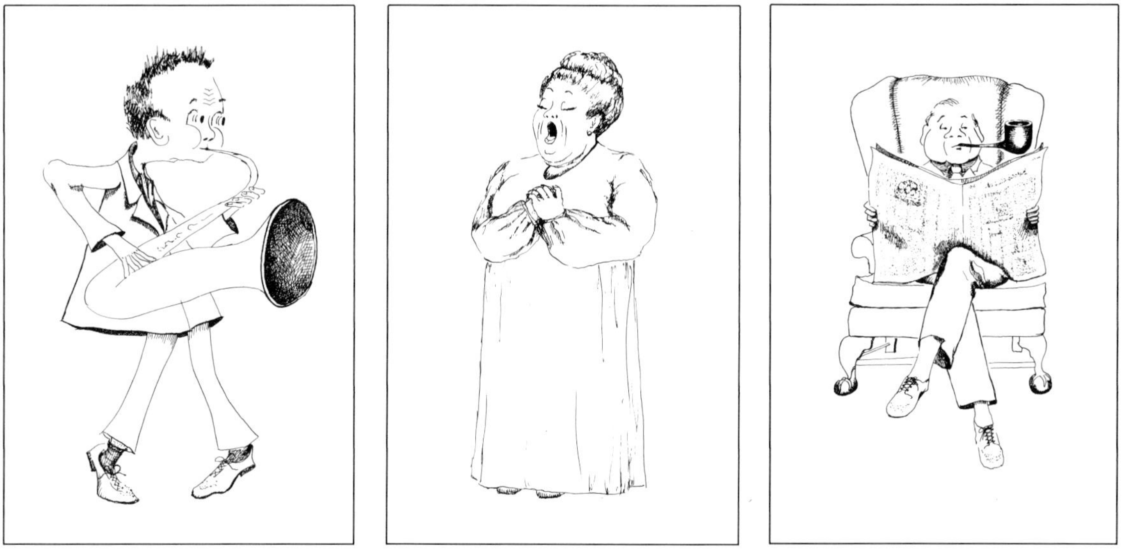

Figs. 1-7a to c Hobbies or occupations of the patient can be affected by the wearing of dentures.

Other patients want their new dentures to help remove wrinkles from their face in order to look younger—a "prosthetic facelift" (Fig. 1-9). We should alert patients that dentures cannot remove all wrinkles and that the plastic surgeon is the person they ought to see.

Sometimes the patient does not have to talk at all because the patient's past and future troubles are manifest by the bagful of dentures he brings to a visit (Fig. 1-10). This patient may be the type not only to complain about the dentures, but also to criticize each dentist who made them. Treat-

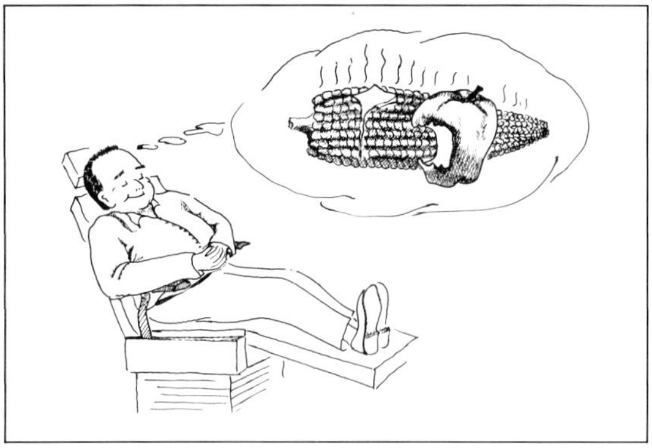

Fig. 1-8 This patient is dreaming about being able to eat corn on the cob and apples, but is this a realistic expectation?

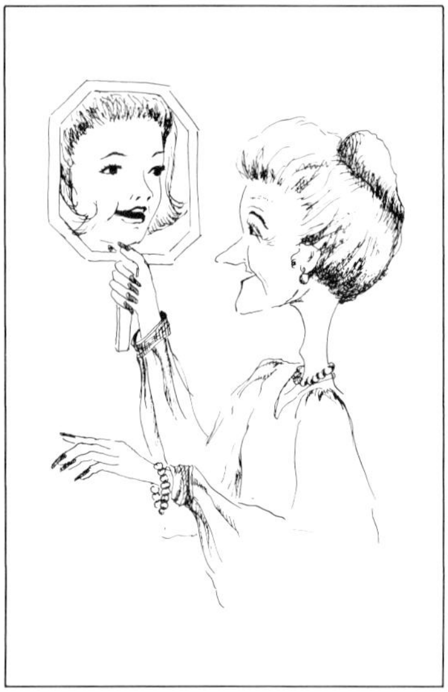

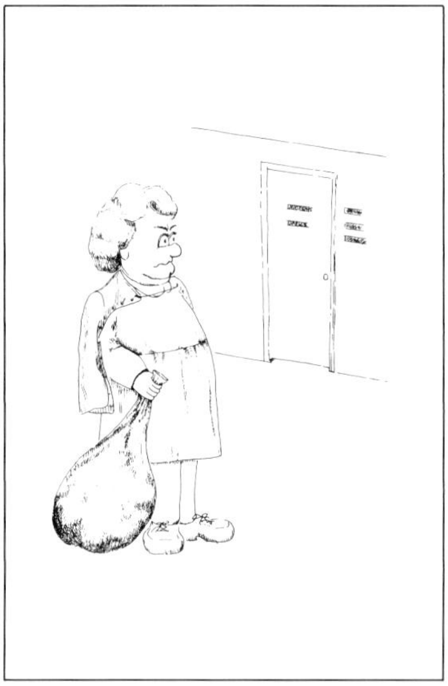

Fig. 1-9 *(left)* This patient has a dream that new dentures can remove wrinkles.

Fig. 1-10 *(right)* This patient's troubles are manifested in the bagful of dentures brought to the first visit.

ment on this patient should not begin until you can communicate directly with the dentists who made them (if possible). If the patient is reluctant to tell you who made them, you should consider not beginning treatment. The other dentist can often reveal to you any problems that he may have had in treating the patient: Did the patient show up for all appointments or were there multiple cancellations? Did the patient pay for the dentures? What was the patient's attitude? *You should refrain from criticizing the work that was done, because you do not know the circumstances under which the work was accomplished.* Without appropriate consultation with the previous dentist(s), you may well be added to this patient's failure list. At the same time, it is important to listen to the patient's complaints as being sincere and real, and to evaluate what changes, if any, could make the patient comfortable and happy.

Socioeconomic factors

Many people in the lower income brackets expect to wear dentures at a relatively early age—often their parents and grandparents did. Some people in the higher income brackets would consider the suggestion that they have their teeth removed an insult and embarrassment. Time and energy must be spent with each group to educate each realistically about their dental needs. Whether dentures are indicated or not, each patient should understand the prospective treatment and the likely prognosis. Many patients believe that dentures will put an end to their previous history of dental problems, but they should understand that, on the contrary, they might be the beginning of years of agony and displeasure.

YMATO factor: You, Me, and All Those Others

When a patient begins treatment we are faced with treating at least two people: *You*—the patient, and *Me*—the dentist. *You*, the patient, may or may not know what you want or expect from the dentures. *Me*, the dentist, may or may not know what I am going to do. By examination and diagnosis and attempting to know each other, we hopefully come to a reasonable treatment plan. The "You" and "Me" form the YM of the YMATO factor.[2]

The rest of the factor, the All Those Others, means all other considerations that are likely to affect the outcome of treatment. Some examples: The dentist may be tired or not feeling well on a particular day, or may be having personal problems at home or at work. The assistant may be upset or not have shown up at work. The dental hygienist just quit. The laboratory technician called to say that the denture broke while being polished. The patient or dentist gets sick for an entire month in the middle of treatment. The patient's wife or husband plays such a personal, involved role in the fabrication of the dentures that it begins to drive the dentist crazy. All these factors and more can affect the result of the work.

Duplicating the patient's existing dentures

It is often tempting to try to adjust a patient's existing dentures before or during the time the new dentures are being made. The patient may even expect you to "fix up" the existing dentures without making new ones. Sometimes the dentures are used to hold tissue conditioning material to treat unhealthy tissues or to make the patient more comfortable temporarily. If the new dentures are not successful, the patient may complain not only that you could not make him new dentures, but that you ruined the old dentures by adjusting or relining them. *Once you touch a patient's existing dentures, even to adjust a sore spot, you may be committed to adjusting them for a long time.*

Inadequate dentures will forever require adjusting—and most likely with no profit. A reasonable alternative is to duplicate the patient's existing dentures and use these to treat tissue and make other diagnostic changes. If the treatment for new dentures is unsuccessful, you have not altered the patient's original dentures, and the patient can continue to wear them without complaining that you made them worse.

Medical, psychological, and behavioral considerations

The medical history and the Cornell Medical Index

Prior to meeting with the dentist, the patient should be asked to complete a medical health history form. The dental assistant should be available to assist patients in completing the form, particularly those patients who have language problems or physical handicaps or who are elderly. Some medical problems may significantly affect both dental care and the prognosis and some dental care may affect certain medical problems. A standard health history form may reveal that a patient has such medical problems as heart disease, diabetes, Parkinson's disease, rheumatic fever, and arthritis. However, such a health history may reveal nothing about behavioral, personality, or emotional disorders that could significantly affect the outcome of dental treatment.

The Cornell Medical Index* is a well-estab-

*Cornell University Medical College, 1300 York Ave., New York, N.Y. 10021-1974.

Table 1-1 Contrasting attitudes toward wearing dentures

Patient with excellent prognosis	Patient with poor prognosis
Not demanding or exacting; quite accommodating	Demanding and exacting; pays attention to small details
Well-balanced life-style; not preoccupied with denture problem	Preoccupied with denture problems; has consulted several other dentists
Motivated to succeed with dentures	Poorly motivated to succeed with dentures
Has realistic expectations for dentures; has successfully worn complete dentures	Has unattainable expectations for dentures; has not successfully worn complete dentures

lished technique of medical history taking that will bring forth possible psychological or behavior problems. The CMI collects its data by asking questions such as:

1. Do you sweat or tremble a lot during examinations or questioning?
2. Do strange people or places make you afraid?
3. Do you feel alone and sad at a party?
4. Do you often cry?
5. Does worrying continually get you down?
6. Are you considered a touchy person?
7. Are you easily upset or irritated?
8. Are you constantly keyed up and jittery?

The 195 questions on the CMI were chosen to correspond closely to those usually asked in a detailed medical interview, which includes many on the psychological and behavioral aspects of the problem. Questions are in simple, nontechnical English and take the patient approximately 20 minutes to complete. After each question a "yes" or "no" is printed and the patient circles the appropriate answer. In every instance a "yes" response indicates that a patient does have the symptoms about which he is being questioned. There are separate questionnaires for men and women with gender-related questions.

An important benefit in using this questionnaire is that you can score and interpret it *before* you meet the patient, allowing you to get to "know" the patient before being introduced. According to the information reported in the CMI instruction manual, if more than 25 "yes" responses are recorded, there is a potential problem. The questionnaire is divided into 18 sections by body systems. If the "yes" responses are located mainly in one or two sections, the patient's problem is likely localized and is of an organic nature. In contrast, if the "yes" responses are scattered throughout all sections of the CMI the medical problem is likely to be generalized, usually involving a psychological or emotional disturbance. Also, if three or more "yes" responses occur in the last page, the possibility of an emotional problem is suggested.

Bolender, Swoope, and Smith used the CMI on a group of 402 dental patients and found a direct relationship between patient satisfaction with new dentures and a score above the critical levels of the CMI score (more than 25 "yes" responses or more than three "yes" responses on the last page of the form).[3] Patient dissatisfaction increased abruptly for those patients who answered "yes" more than six times on the last page. This group of patients was accepted for treatment only after discussing the relationship of their emotional problems and dental problem. (The term "nervous" was substituted for "emotional" when discussing this with the patient.) These patients were forewarned that they should expect difficulty in adjusting to new dentures.

Attitude

The patient's attitudes toward wearing some sort of removable prosthesis must be determined. A pa-

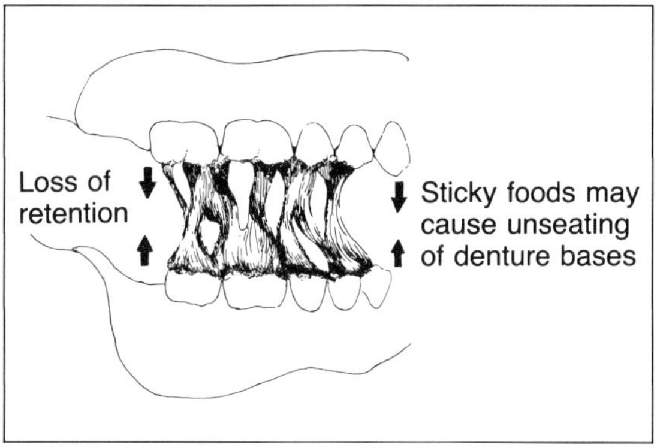

Fig. 1-11a Retention is the resistance to dislodgement.

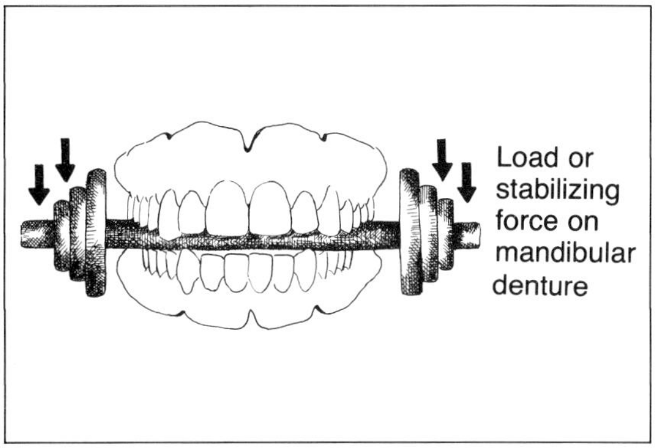

Fig. 1-11b Stability is the resistance to a load placed upon the prosthesis.

tient may fall anywhere between two extremes in behavior (Table 1-1). The patient's previous denture experience may contribute to his attitude. The patient who previously was unsuccessful in wearing dentures may have a poor attitude, whereas the patient who was happy with previous dentures may carry a better attitude toward new dentures.

Anatomic and physiologic factors

The degree of success with which complete dentures can be made for a patient is based also upon the anatomy of the edentulous maxilla and mandible. A thorough understanding of the patient's denture as related to the anatomy and to the health of the tissues helps to determine a prognosis. The principles and techniques of making impressions that are described later in this book are based on the concepts of how to utilize the patient's existing anatomy and behavioral factors to achieve the most stability, retention, esthetics, and patient comfort and to therefore achieve the best prognosis and results.

A thorough visual and digital examination is done of the entire oral cavity, including the cheeks and lips, to ensure that a complete oral cancer screening is included. Inflammatory or pathologic changes may exist in response to the patient's existing dentures. For example, examination may reveal papillary hyperplasia, denture stomatitis, or hyperplastic tissue. Bony exostoses, undercuts, or sharp ridges may be present to complicate treatment. A decision must be made whether or not to treat or first perform preprosthetic surgery on the existing tissue conditions.

The mandibular prognosis

The prognosis for a mandibular complete denture can be divided into the factors which affect stability and the factors which affect retention. *Retention* is that quality inherent in the prosthesis which resists the force of gravity and the adhesiveness of foods (Fig. 1-11a). *Stability* is the resistance of a denture base to movement under an occlusal load (Fig. 1-11b).

The retention and stability achieved by a denture can differ from patient to patient and are dependent upon both the anatomic and physiologic features that exist. Tables 1-2 and 1-3 outline the factors that affect retention and stability and assign a numerical value to each, a more specific application of the prognosis rating scale described earlier.

The highly resorbed mandibular ridge

The first thing that most dentists look at is the amount of residual ridge bone that remains. If not much bone is remaining, the immediate assumption is that it will be very difficult to make a successful mandibular denture. *Most dentists don't investigate any further.* They automatically decide that the patient won't be able to wear mandibular

Table 1-2 Anatomic prognosis for a mandibular complete denture, retention criteria

Factors	Criteria for retention: Best prognosis (1)	Criteria for retention: Worst prognosis (3)
Nature of sublingual fold space (SLFS)	Defined SLFS	Sloping, draping floor of mouth; no definition to SLFS
Tongue position (based on Wright's[4] classification)	Normal (tip lies just lingual to anterior teeth)	Retracted
Position of buccal fat pad	Rests on the masseteric notch area of the denture	Does not rest on masseteric notch area
Tissue tonicity	Cheek and lip tissue full and resilient	Cheek and lip tissue tense and taut
Denture-bearing tissue	Firm, definite cushion of mucosa	Thin, inelastic mucosa
Amount of interarch space at vertical dimension of occlusion	Adequate: entire denture-bearing area is covered	Inadequate: surgery is contraindicated

Table 1-3 Anatomic prognosis for a mandibular complete denture, stability criteria

Factors	Criteria for stability: Best prognosis (1)	Criteria for stability: Worst prognosis (3)
Buccal shelf supporting area	Flat and broad	Sloping, narrow, or concave
Tongue position (based on Wright's[4] classification)	Normal (tip lies just lingual to anterior teeth)	Retracted
Position of buccal fat pad	Rests on the masseteric notch	Does not rest on the masseteric notch
Tissue tonicity	Cheek and lip tissue full and resilient	Cheek and lip tissue tense and taut
Denture-bearing tissue	Firm, connective tissue support	Redundant, movable tissue or thin, inelastic mucosa
Amount of interarch space at vertical dimension of occlusion	Adequate: entire denture-bearing area is covered	Inadequate: surgery is contraindicated

Table 1-4 Anatomic prognosis for a maxillary complete denture, retention and stability criteria

Factors	Criteria for retention and stability: Best prognosis (1)	Criteria for retention and stability: Worst prognosis (3)
Ridge form	Broad, U-shaped or flat; nonundercut	Deep, V-shaped vault; undercuts
Vestibular extensions	Resilient, displaceable mucosa with depth	Taut, tense, shallow vestibule
Denture-bearing tissues	Firm, definite cushion of submucosa	Thin, inelastic mucosa

dentures successfully and consider referring the patient to a specialist. As was stated earlier, 70% of all denture patients can be treated successfully without much difficulty. A good number of patients who make up this 70% group have significantly resorbed mandibular ridges, yet they wear the mandibular denture without a problem. It is important to know that a high, well-formed mandibular ridge is *not* always needed for denture success. Oral surgeons often perform ridge augmentation procedures and vestibular extension to increase the height of the mandibular ridge. Yet this increased ridge height does not necessarily improve the prognosis for wearing dentures. In fact, a resorbed ridge often leaves more room to set teeth without significantly decreasing the stability or retention.

Other anatomic factors to consider that do enhance the prognosis are the character of the sublingual fold space, the tongue position, the nature of the buccal shelf, the form and position of the buccal fat pad, and the tonicity of the denture-bearing tissues (Tables 1-2 to 1-4). Each factor will be discussed and illustrated separately as it relates to the prognosis.

Anatomic factors affecting mandibular denture prognosis

Sublingual fold space. This is the potential space that lies between the lower anterior ridge and the sublingual gland (Fig. 1-12). The denture base border extension lies within this space. The sublingual fold space can assume many anatomic forms and can be divided into two distinct categories—well defined and poorly defined—with many variations possible between.

In a *well-defined* sublingual fold space the space is clearly evident and delineated between the mandibular anterior ridge and the sublingual gland. A seal of the denture base extension can be achieved in this area when the tissues of the gland that lie posteriorly to the denture rest upon the periphery of the denture base (Fig. 1-13).

An overall peripheral seal is extremely important in this location and is the objective to be attained. The seal should be thought of as extending around all peripheral areas of the denture base. This concept usually is spoken of only in reference to the maxillary denture base. The level of the floor of the mouth in this region is mainly dependent upon the activity of the genioglossus muscle (Fig. 1-14).

The genioglossus muscle lies superior to the geniohyoid and mylohyoid muscles in the region and, because of its activity, can play a significant role as to the character of this anatomic area. Tongue movement posteriorly, caused by the contraction of the genioglossus muscle, plays a critical role in the anatomic form that the sublingual fold space will have. As the tongue moves posteriorly, it carries the tissues of the sublingual gland with it to take away the posterior border of the sublingual fold space. This will be discussed in greater detail in a later chapter. The mylohyoid muscle has little

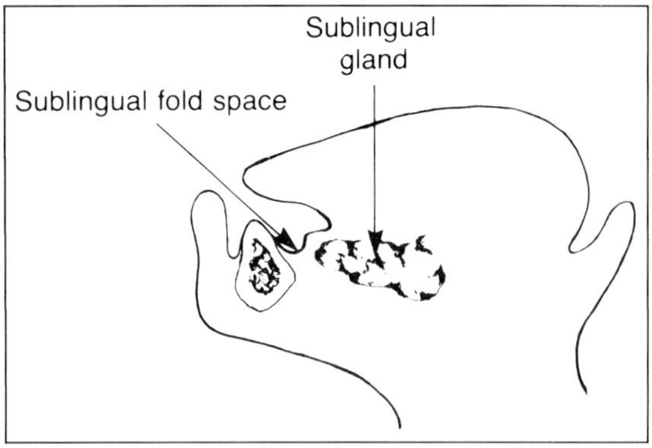

Fig. 1-12 The sublingual fold space is the potential space that lies between the mandibular anterior ridge and the tissues of the sublingual gland.

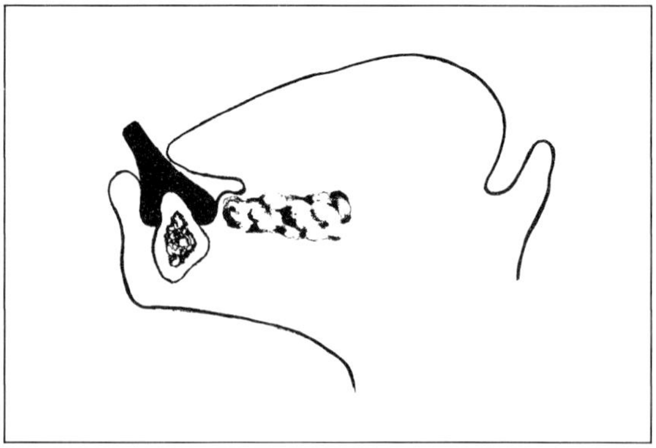

Fig. 1-13 An acrylic resin impression tray and impression material will fill up the space between the ridge and the sublingual fold. This is the sublingual fold space.

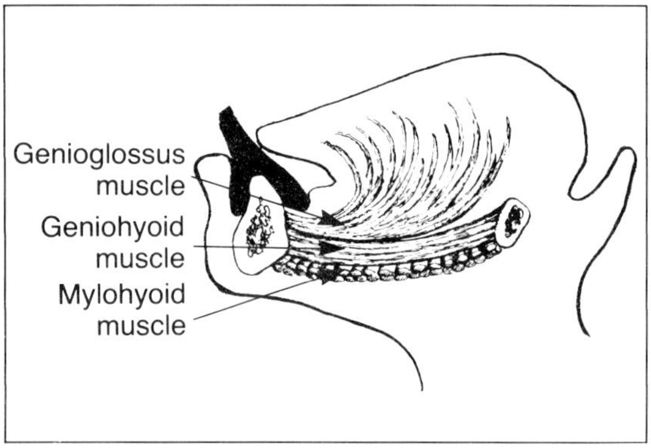

Fig. 1-14 The level of the floor of the mouth in the sublingual fold space area is dependent mainly upon the activity of the genioglossus muscle.

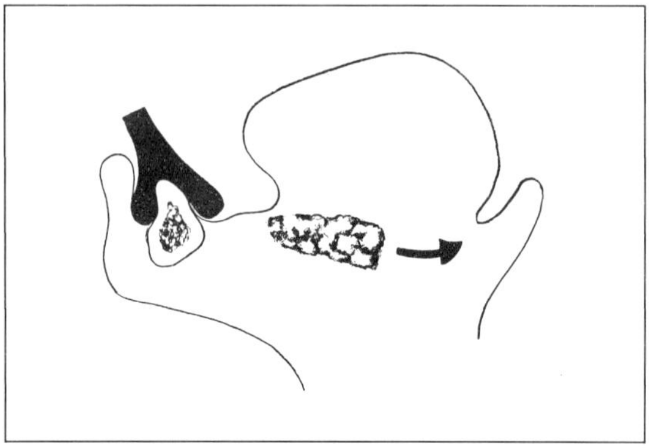

Fig. 1-15a A poorly defined sublingual fold space occurs where the sublingual gland tissues are drawn posteriorly *(arrow)* and therefore are not present to seal the denture in this region.

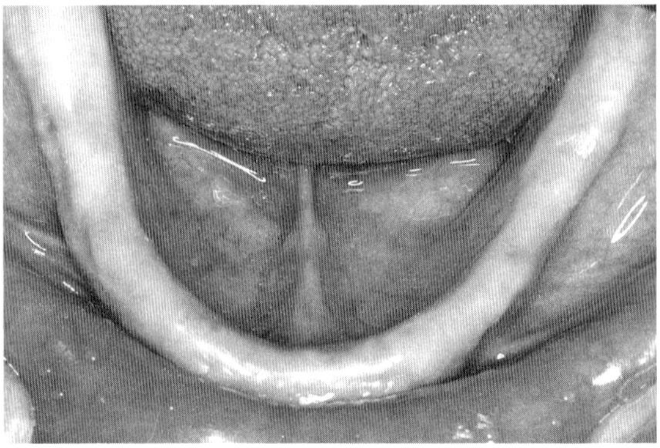

Fig. 1-15b The tongue rests posteriorly and therefore is not present to seal the denture base in this area.

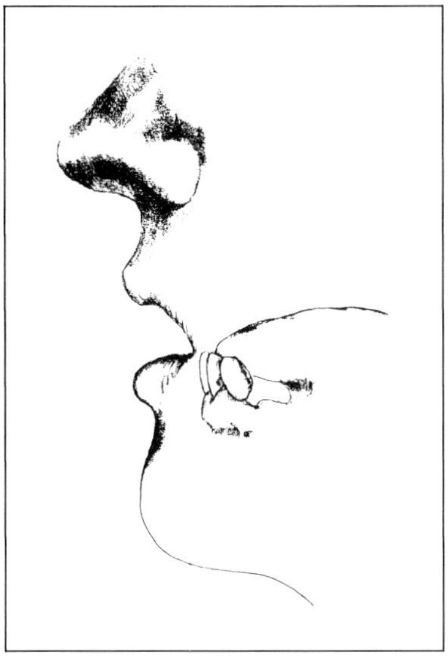

Fig. 1-16a *(left)* A normal tongue position occurs when the tip of the tongue rests upon the lingual aspect of the mandibular anterior teeth.

Fig. 1-16b *(below)* Frontal view of normal tongue position.

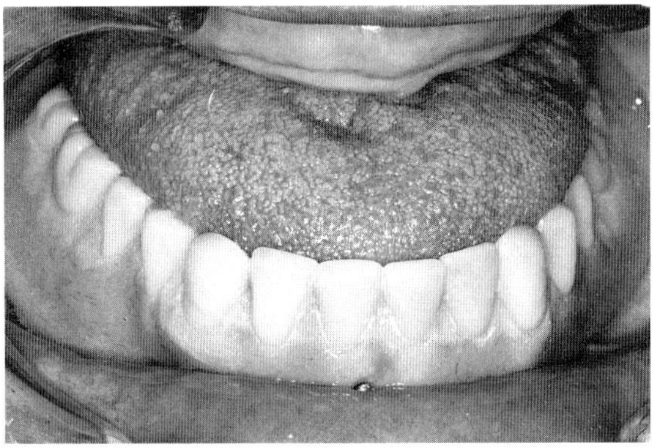

effect upon this region because of its inferior position in relation to the other tissues.

In a *poorly defined* sublingual fold space the sublingual gland tissues are absent or are drawn posteriorly and therefore are not present to "seal" the denture in this region (Figs. 1-15a and b). One cannot expect to attain as much overall retention in this situation because the peripheral seal is now absent. This situation is referred to as a draping floor of the mouth.

Tongue position. This is the position that the tongue assumes at rest and during function. It plays an important role in the anatomic form that the sublingual fold space will assume. A *normal* tongue position, as Wright defines it, is one where the tip (apex) of the tongue rests forward in a position just lingual to the mandibular anterior teeth[4] (Figs. 1-16a and b). In this situation the sublingual gland and its overlying tissues are drawn forward to aid in sealing the denture flange in the sublingual fold space by maintaining contact with it. Wright states that 65% of all patients have a normal tongue position.[4]

A *retracted* tongue position (which includes the remaining 35% of the patients) causes the tissues of the sublingual gland to move posteriorly and inferiorly to break the seal between the mucous membranes overlying the sublingual gland and the denture periphery (Fig. 1-17). Without this tissue-denture border contact, a seal is not achieved and retention is sacrificed.

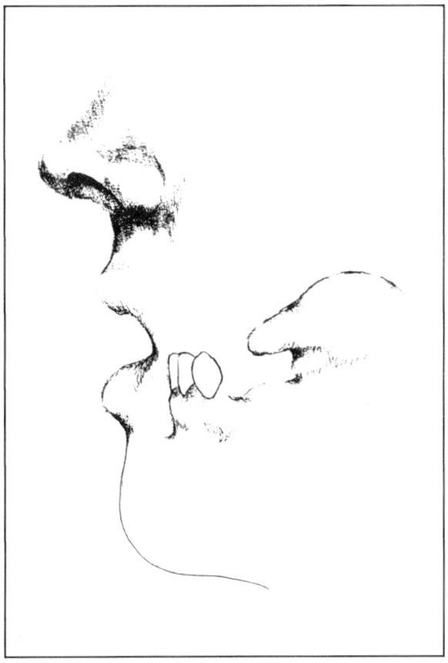

Fig. 1-17 A retracted tongue position occurs when the tip of the tongue is drawn posteriorly. This causes the tissues of the sublingual gland to move with it.

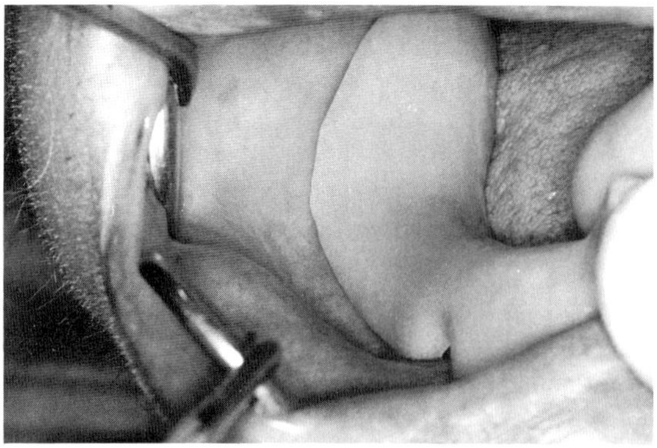

Fig. 1-18a The buccal fat pad is retracted back with the mirror head.

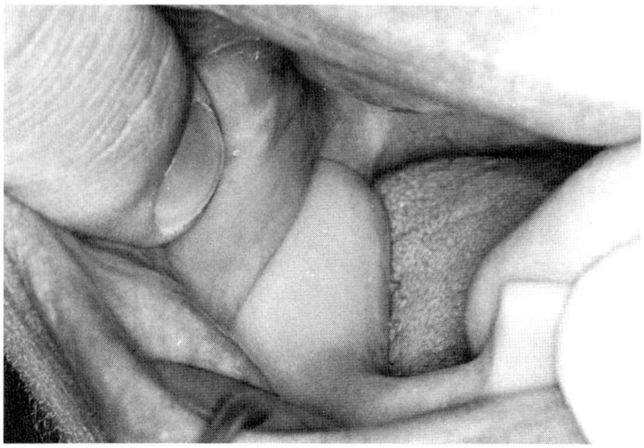

Fig. 1-18b The buccal fat pad rests upon the masseteric notch area of the impression tray. This ultimately aids in stability and retention of the denture base.

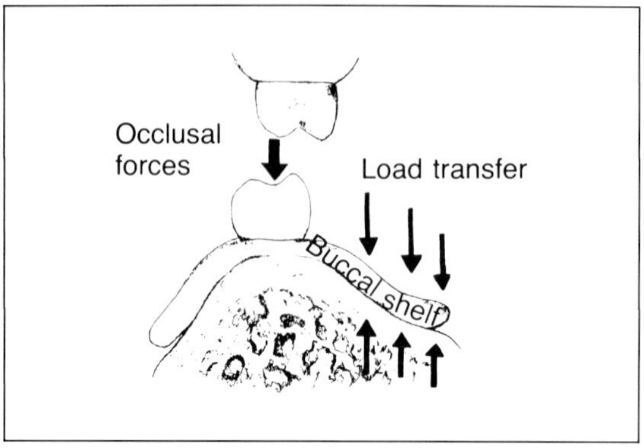

Fig. 1-19 A broad, flat buccal shelf can offer good support to the occlusal forces that are placed upon the denture base.

Buccal fat pad. The buccal fat pad is the pad of areolar connective tissues that lies within the posterior cheek. It lies in the vicinity of the masseteric notch area of the denture base. This pad of tissue can be beneficial to both retention and stability. It aids in retention if it rests upon the denture border of the masseteric notch area to achieve a seal, and it helps in stabilizing the denture base by resting upon it (Figs. 1-18a and b).

Tonicity of the tissue. Tonicity is the relative resiliency or tautness of the cheek and lip tissue. If the tissues are tense and taut, there can be a tendency for the denture base to lift off its basal seat, therefore affecting retention. This is particularly true if the denture bases are overextended. If the tissues are taut, it may be difficult to maintain a seat to the denture, therefore affecting stability. If the tissues that lie directly beneath the denture base are redundant and movable, this will affect the stability of the denture. When the denture is in function the tissue will be more easily displaced and the denture will move with it.

The opposite can occur where the supporting tissues are thin and inelastic in nature. The mucosa in this situation lacks the "cushion" effect of a thicker mucosa. This can allow the denture to move and slide more easily. Retention may be partially affected in that if a cushion of mucosa does not exist, a seal of the denture borders to the adjacent tissue is not as effectively accomplished.

Buccal shelf. The buccal shelf is the key to the stability of the mandibular denture because of its large surface area of support. Although all the slopes of the mandibular ridges are important for support, the buccal shelf is particularly significant because when it is broad and flat it can offer the best support and resistance to occlusal forces (Fig. 1-19). A sharply sloping, narrow, or concave buccal shelf would not offer the same support because of its shape and size.

Interarch distance. The availability of room to place the maxillary and mandibular denture bases and teeth is routinely evaluated at the first diagnostic visit. An easy way to evaluate this is to place your thumb between the maxillary and mandibular

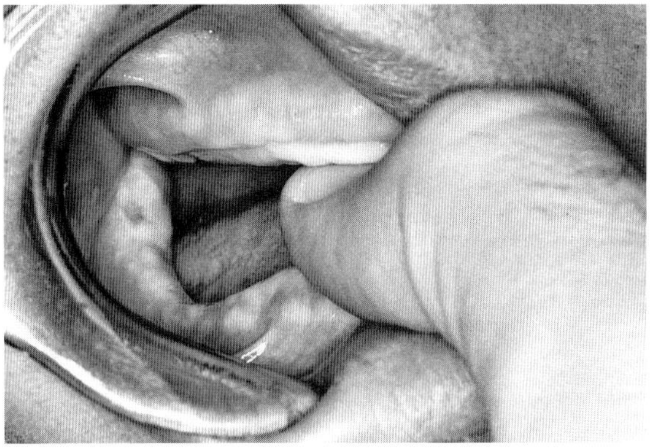

Fig. 1-20 The dentist's thumb is placed between the anterior ridges and the patient is instructed to close his mouth. This gives a rough estimate of the amount of room available posteriorly.

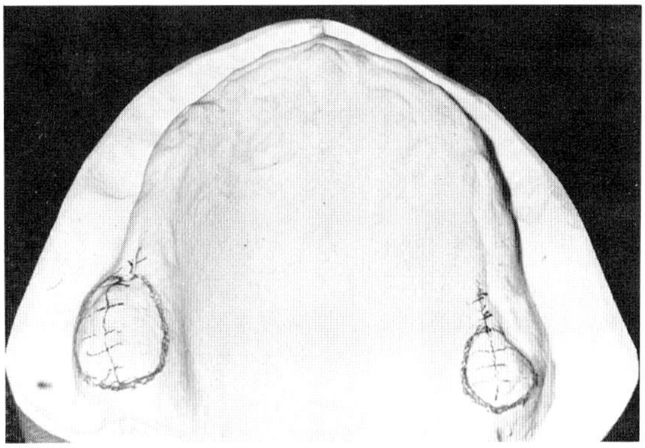

Fig. 1-21 Diagnostic casts are sent to the oral surgeon to indicate how much reduction is required for adequate dentures to be made.

anterior ridges and instruct the patient to close against your thumb. The cheeks are then reflected open on each side to inspect the amount of available room (Fig. 1-20). If you suspect that there may not be enough room, it is important to do a diagnostic mounting of casts at the expected vertical dimension of occlusion.

It also helps to examine the patient's existing dentures. Often the distal extensions of the mandibular denture base do not cover the pear-shaped pad because of this lack of room posteriorly. It is useful to evaluate the vertical dimension of occlusion with these existing dentures. If the vertical dimension of occlusion is correct, then a tuberosity reduction is most likely indicated. It might be best to refer the patient to an oral surgeon for reduction of the maxillary tuberosity or other ridge areas to make room. Diagnostic casts can be used to outline the amount of reduction that is needed (Fig. 1-21).

These casts are a tremendous help to the oral surgeon who usually, at the time of surgery, wonders how much reduction is really needed. Without such casts, inadequate reduction is often accomplished and a second or third surgery has to be performed at a later date. If the entire desired denture-bearing area in either arch is not covered, this could adversely affect the amount of retention and stability that will be achieved.

Maxillary prognosis

The prognosis for the maxillary complete denture also can be divided into factors that can affect stability and retention. The maxillary denture does not generally present the same problems in stability or retention as a mandibular denture because of the obvious anatomical difference. The availability and excellence of the peripheral seal and the broad, continuous surface area connecting the entire denture periphery make the maxillary denture the more retentive and stable. The factors listed in Table 1-4 are similar to those discussed in Tables 1-2 and 1-3 for the mandible, with the exception of the ridge form. A broad, U-shaped or flat ridge offers good support, while a narrow, V-shaped, high palate offers poor support.

Conclusion

Keep in mind that the examination, diagnostic, and prognostic phase of complete denture fabrication may be accomplished in one short visit for some patients, while it may take several visits for others. As mentioned earlier, for some patients you may have to make transitional or diagnostic dentures to determine the prognosis or the feasibility of continuing treatment. With these patients, it is important to not make a commitment to treatment until you complete the appropriate diagnostic procedures and determine the prognosis. With all patients, it is important to give this phase of treatment the time and attention your patient deserves.

References

1. Brewer, A.A., and Morrow, R.M. Overdentures. St. Louis: C.V. Mosby Co., 1980.
2. Brewer, A.A. Selection of denture teeth for esthetics and function. J. Prosthet. Dent. 23:371, 1970.
3. Bolender, C.L., Swoope, C.C., and Smith, D.E. The Cornell Medical Index as a prognostic aid for complete dentures. J. Prosthet. Dent. 22:20, 1969.
4. Wright, C.R. A study of the tongue and its relation to denture stability. J. Am. Dent. Assoc. 39:269, 1949.

Early in my practice I found it very disconcerting to have failures. This was hard on my ego. These failures were most evident when complete dentures were constructed. Therefore, I set about learning all I could about complete dentures. I read every book and article on complete dentures that I could lay my hands on. I enrolled in many courses, and used every face-bow and hinge-bow I could obtain; worked with almost every articulator that had been produced; used many impression techniques and many different types of teeth. I even made hinge-bows, articulators, centric relation recording devices, and teeth of my own. I spent 5 years in dental research, much of it trying to find out how teeth contacted in mastication and in other functions. My percentage of failures decreased. I found that once I had refined my mechanical skills I was able to construct successful dentures, regardless of the technique or instruments used. But, I still had failures. Today I have no failures. This was accomplished in two ways. First, I rearranged my thinking—I no longer have failures, but I have varying degrees of success. Second, and more important, I treat the patient instead of just constructing dentures for him. The two principal personalities concerned in complete denture service, the dentist and the patient, are thus immediately more comfortable.

Allen Brewer

(From: Treating complete denture patients. J. Prosthet. Dent. 14:1015, 1016, 1964.)

Chapter 2

Philosophy of Impression Making

The primary objective of making an impression of an edentulous arch is to produce a denture base that will be stable, retentive, comfortable, and esthetic and that will preserve the remaining tissues.

Over the past decades the different philosophies and techniques of impression making have been a major controversy in dentistry. Unfortunately, the science of impression making is still in the philosophical stage because definitive research to tell us which techniques are the best is not available.

The controversy has centered around *(1)* the amount of pressure applied to the tissues while making the impression, *(2)* the degree of tissue detail that is captured, *(3)* the type of impression material selected, *(4)* the type of impression tray used, *(5)* whether the mouth is open or closed when the impression is made, and *(6)* whether the peripheral borders of the denture are functionally border molded or arbitrarily located.

According to Devan, the difficulty in making edentulous impressions is due to the fact that the mouth is lined with tissue of varying displaceability.[1] The amount of tissue displaceability varies according to the tissue's thickness, its rigidity, the forces applied to it, and its anatomic location in the mouth.

We are not making impressions of a mannequin. Tissue tone varies from patient to patient and from one area of the mouth to another. As you can imagine, applying the same force to each anatomic area of the mouth will cause many different responses in movement of the tissues. The forces directed to the tissues during impression making can be increased or decreased by altering the *(1)* viscosity and flow of the impression material used, *(2)* type of impression tray made, and *(3)* forces exerted upon the tray when the impression is being made.

Discussion continues to focus on whether impressions of the denture-bearing (supporting) tissues should be made in the resting, unloaded form or under some increased load to simulate a functional state. Some techniques use minimal tissue placement, while others advocate using a significant amount of pressure. There are also methods that selectively apply more pressure to certain anatomic areas than others. These are referred to as selective tissue placement techniques (Fig. 2-1).

Minimal pressure techniques

The primary objective of making a minimal pressure impression is to make the impression without displacing the tissues, therefore capturing them in their most undisturbed state. An impression material of low viscosity and high flow capabilities is selected, and a minimal amount of pressure is used in seating and holding the impression tray.

These techniques are advocated for two reasons. First, the dentures are under pressure from occlusal load only a relatively small amount of time, so the dentures should fit this relaxed, unloaded tissue surface. Second, it has been suggested that if the tissues are recorded in an undisturbed state with a very accurate, free-flowing impression material, retention and stability of the dentures will be in-

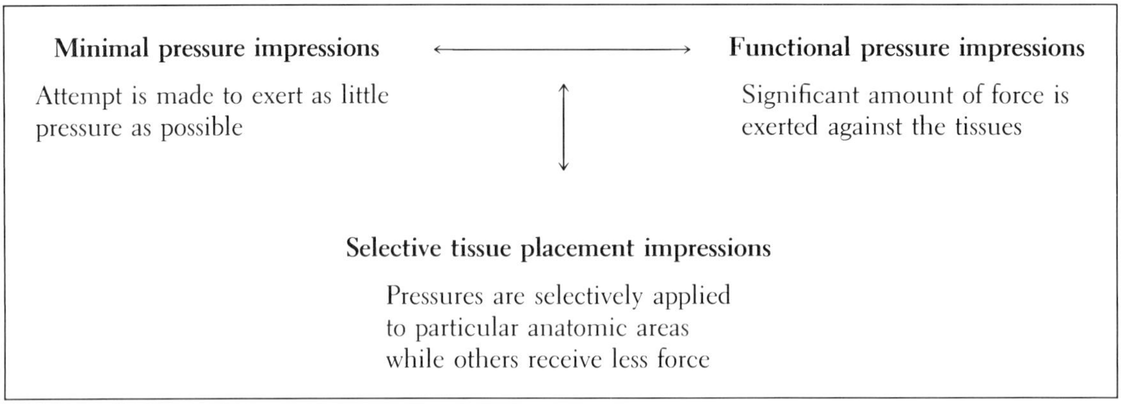

Fig. 2-1 Classification of impression making by the forces that are applied.

creased. This belief is based upon the mucostatic technique as described by Page.[2] Page believed that if the denture bases were perfectly adapted to the edentulous tissues, then the surface tension of the saliva layer between the denture and tissue would be so strong that the denture could not be removed without a great deal of force. Denen advocated an impression technique using alginate because he felt that the material and his technique were so static that they exerted a "negative pressure."[3] Sharry stated that "nonpressure" and "negative pressure" techniques do not exist.[4] Rather, these are semantic devices used to dramatize the minimal amount of force desirable in making impressions.

Pressure techniques

At the opposite extreme, a pressure impression is one in which an impression of the tissues is purposely made under a significant load. In this situation, the impression material and the tray that supports it are less displaceable than the tissue. The operator applies force in seating the impression tray and/or asks the patient to close his mouth with force while the impression material sets. Pressure techniques produce final casts in which the tissue has been displaced significantly more than with a nonpressure technique. Pressure impressions are made to simulate the position that the tissue will assume when the completed denture is under a functional load. The logic here is that if the same force can be used against the tissue as is used, for example, during chewing, there would be more intimacy of tissue–denture base contact during function and therefore a more stable denture. This increased tissue contact would allow for less play of the denture under occlusal load. The tissues would already be displaced or under load by the denture base before occlusal contact were made. This tissue load would displace the tissues closer to the underlying bone, which would then offer firm support to the denture. Opponents of pressure impression techniques believe that *(1)* the displaced soft tissues tend to rebound upon the denture base when the patient is at rest, providing a constant dislodging force, and *(2)* the increased pressure causes tissue compression beyond its biologic tolerance, resulting tissue irritation, and potentially increased bone resorption.

Selective tissue placement technique

A selective tissue placement technique is one in which the dentist can decide which denture-bearing tissues to make impressions of with more or less tissue placement. A selective placement impression is used to record some tissues in a relaxed, relatively unaltered state and other tissues with a determined amount of placement. The purpose is to best utilize the patient's particular anatomy and tissue tone to achieve the most stability and retention. This technique takes into consideration the differences in tissue tone and displaceability.

According to Sears, we do not *take* impressions as we would on a mannequin; rather, we *make* impressions to accommodate the tissues with their various degrees of displaceability and form.[5] By knowing a particular patient's anatomy and tissue tone, the dentist can select an impression technique to create results that meet his objectives for stability, retention, and patient comfort. As Devan said, the ideal impression must be in the mind of the dentist before it can be in his hand (Fig. 2-2).[1]

The technique of impression making as described in this book begins with a preliminary alginate impression made in a stock edentulous tray. The quality of this impression is as important as that of the final impression. If the denture-bearing area is not captured in its entirety, the custom acrylic resin tray that is made from it will be inadequate. The preliminary alginate impression is made and then trimmed to closely resemble the completed denture form in both border height and width. A custom acrylic resin impression tray with peripheral relief is used to make a selective tissue placement impression. This custom tray offers a means by which the dentist can control the amount and location of tissue placement applied to the denture-bearing tissues while the final impression is being made. The principle of selective tissue placement is applied here, because the alginate impression material records the attached mucosa with minimal placement, while compound records the more movable tissues and peripheral sulcus areas with additional placement. The slopes of the ridges are primary supporting areas, and they are functionally loaded during the final impression process. The compound on the slopes of the ridges pushes the movable mucosa closer to its underlying bony support. Therefore, the final denture base will selectively apply additional placement of these tissues. The ridge crest areas (the areas of attached gingiva) will therefore receive less placement when the denture is in function.

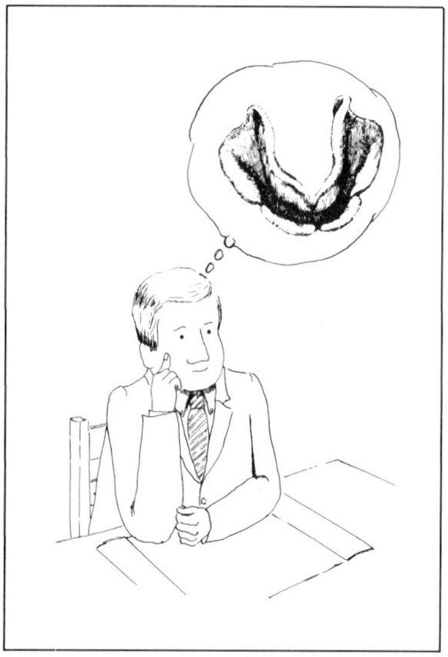

Fig. 2-2 The impression must be in the mind of the dentist before it can be in hand. It is this knowledge and experience that enable a dentist to create desirable results.

References

1. Devan, M.M. Basic principles of impression making. J. Prosthet. Dent. 2:26, 1952.
2. Page, H.L. Mucostatics—a principle not a technique. Chicago, 1946. Published personally by Harry L. Page, 1625 East Washington St., Chicago, Ill.
3. Denen, H.E. Negative pressure impressions for full dentures. J. Am. Dent. Assoc. 31:888, 1944.
4. Sharry, J. Complete denture prosthodontics. pp. 169–186 *In* Theories of Impressions. New York: McGraw-Hill, 1962.
5. Sears, V.H. Functional impressions for rebasing full dentures. J. Am. Dent. Assoc. 23:1031, 1936.

In any endeavor we undertake, a smooth road to success is usually the result of good planning. It is seldom luck. We can compare our role with a consulting patient to the role of an architect with a prospective home builder. The architect knows that his client could have gone to a builder and said, "Build me a house." The result would be a house commensurate with the builder's ideas of what a house should be. Those of us who have been through this know that the services of a good architect are worth every penny we pay. The architect knows that his client has come to him for advice and help to obtain something that suits him. The good architect then proceeds to find out something of the personality of his client, his needs, desires, and aspirations. Is this to be a short-time residence or a life-time one? Only after he has all the information possible does he start to plan and then to build the house. He plans for utility, beauty, and ease of maintenance; and he supervises every step of construction. He must keep abreast of the development of new materials and techniques in order to provide the optimum service for his client at minimum cost. Many of us are prone to assume the role of the builder. This may be because this is what we spend so much of our time doing—building and rebuilding. This is most true in this age of specialization when frequently we see only within the confines of our own specialty. Unless we are willing to assume our role as architect and plan with our patients, we are going to send more and more of them to the "builder" or illegal practitioner.

Allen Brewer
(From: Treating complete denture patients.
J. Prosthet. Dent. 14:1016, 1964.)

Chapter 3

Preliminary Alginate Impressions

Preliminary impressions are as important as final impressions. An accurate preliminary alginate impression helps to control the accuracy of the remaining impression procedures. The preliminary impression must capture the denture-bearing area in its entirety in order to make an adequate acrylic resin tray from it. The peripheral borders must be accurate in both height and width for the custom tray to be properly extended. If the preliminary impression is accurately made and trimmed, the amount of trimming on the custom tray will be greatly minimized. The completed preliminary impression must closely resemble the eventual denture base.

A custom impression tray is made from the cast of the alginate impression. The custom impression tray borders must be within 3 mm of the desired periphery of the eventual denture border to properly support compound for border molding. If a custom impression tray is underextended in height or width, it will be nearly impossible and quite time consuming to mold compound to adequately capture the peripheral areas.

General considerations for making an alginate impression

Preliminary impressions for the maxilla and mandible are made in stock edentulous-style trays. It is important not to attempt to extend or modify the tray with any strips of soft beading or utility wax. Soft wax added to a tray can adversely affect the impression in several ways. First, the soft wax actively interrupts the flow of the alginate impression material so that the peripheral borders are not captured in their natural form. Second, added wax will usually cause an overextension of a peripheral border in height or width; therefore, the resulting impression will not be accurate. Third, it is common to have "show through" of peripheral wax in the impression. The show through does not represent an accurate impression. Fourth, the added wax offers little support to the alginate as it sets or when it is withdrawn from the mouth. Without firm support, the alginate easily undergoes dimensional change. If the stock tray must be altered, it should be done with compound that, when set, will be hard, will adhere securely to the tray, and will offer the needed support to the alginate.

Room temperature water is used when mixing the alginate impression material. A thermometer can be placed in the water bottle so that the water temperature is seen prior to mixing. Room temperature water is used so that each time a mix is made, the working and setting times of the alginate are consistent. Colder water increases the amount of working time, while hotter water decreases the working time. The problem with using water temperature to alter the setting is not knowing precisely the working and setting time for each impression. Very cold water used to mix the material may cause the material to continue flowing in the patient's mouth when the initial set should have begun. Ideally, the material should stop flowing and begin to set after the loaded tray has been placed in the mouth and seated and positioning has been completed, as will be discussed.

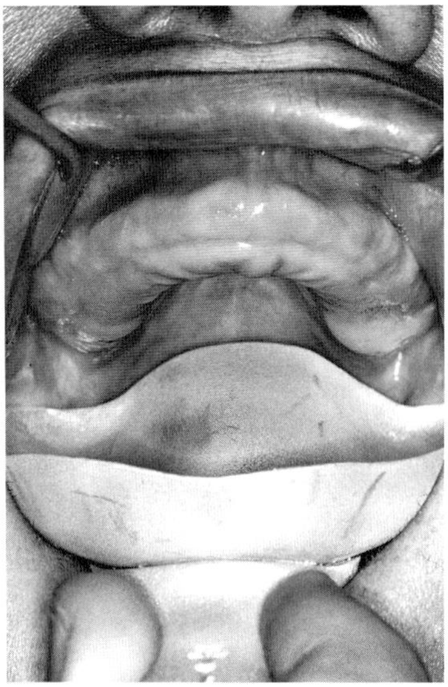

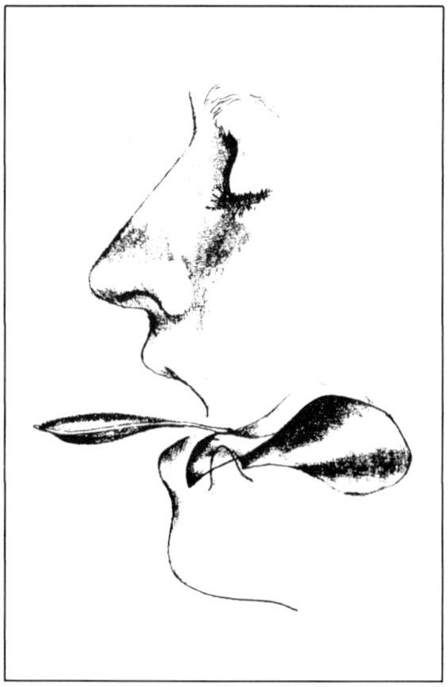

Fig. 3-1 *(left)* To check the adequacy of the impression tray, first seat it posteriorly to cover the most distal areas. Then seat the tray anteriorly—it should cover the anterior ridge, and the flange of the tray should extend into the labial vestibule.

Fig. 3-2 *(right)* A space of approximately one quarter inch should exist between the edentulous ridge and the impression tray.

Either prepackaged alginate or bulk packaged material can be used. If a large can of alginate impression material is opened and not used promptly, it can be weighed in increments for individual impressions and sealed in packages or jars. After a can is opened, it is subjected to atmospheric contaminants and moisture, which can affect its physical properties during later use.

Stone for pouring the cast should be weighed prior to making the impression so that the impression can be poured without delay. A delay of more than ten minutes in pouring an alginate impression can cause significant dimensional change.

Technique

Rehearse with the patient the procedures that will be used to make the impression. Instruct the patient to rinse his mouth vigorously with cold water and then to hold some additional cold water in his mouth until the impression is ready to be made. Ask the patient to either expectorate or swallow the water before the impression is made. Rinsing with cold water dilutes and minimizes saliva buildup and also cools the tissues so that alginate that is manually placed does not set too quickly when it contacts the tissue. Moist labial and buccal tissues enable the peripheral borders to be formed with manual manipulation. If cheeks and lips are dry, the alginate material sticks to the tissues, making manipulation difficult.

Tray selection

Iden Dental* trays are recommended because the mandibular trays have much longer extensions in the retromylohyoid area than other edentulous-style trays. This area is commonly missed in preliminary impressions because the tongue blocks access of the alginate. If the stock tray is short in this area, alginate is not supported to the desired full extension.

The selected tray must be large enough to cover the entire denture-bearing area to be impressioned. Maxillary and mandibular impression trays are selected in the following manner:

1. Select a tray that you think will adequately cover all areas.

*Iden Dental Mfg., Dayton, Ohio.

2. Insert the tray into the mouth and verify its fit.
3. Seat the tray posteriorly first to cover the most distal area that is to be impressioned (Fig. 3-1).
4. Continue to seat the tray anteriorly. Lift the lip and cheek out. The tray should cover the anterior ridge and there should be space between the ridge and the inner surface of the tray (Fig. 3-2). The trays can be removed from the mouth and bent slightly with finger pressure to accommodate anatomic variations.

Mixing the alginate

The armamentarium required for mixing the alginate is *(1)* a large rubber mixing bowl, *(2)* a flexible mixing spatula, *(3)* a thermometer placed in room temperature water, *(4)* a water measure for the alginate, *(5)* premeasured or prepackaged alginate powder (Jeltrate Normal Set, Type II*) and *(6)* a watch or clock with a second hand.

Procedure

1. Place the premeasured amount of water into the mixing bowl. Using slightly less water than powder makes a working consistency that is easy to control and manipulate, especially when using an unaltered stock edentulous-style tray. If the mix is too thin, the alginate will flow uncontrollably.

2. Add the premeasured alginate to the water—not vice versa—to minimize the entrapment of air. Add all of the alginate at once rather than a scoop at a time to avoid having the first scoop begin gelation before the last scoop.

3. Mix vigorously for 45 seconds, forcing the material against the sides of the bowl with the large flexible spatula to eliminate bubbles. Mix in one direction only to prevent incorporating air into the mix. (*Note:* Mechanical spatulation under vacuum is also acceptable. The results are excellent and consistent.)

4. Load the impression tray.

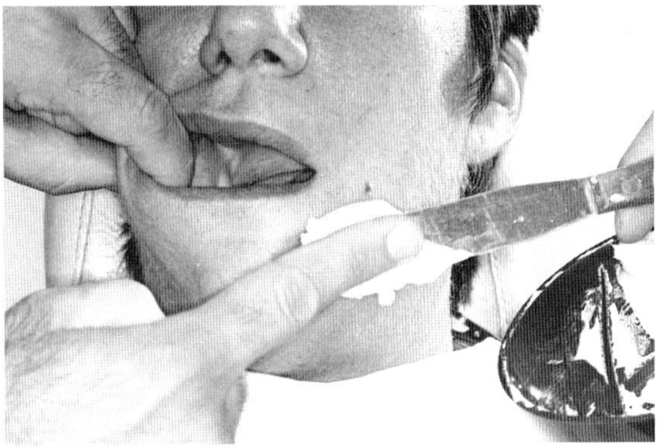

Fig. 3-3 The spatula with a small amount of alginate is held by the assistant. This makes it easy for the dentist to place material in the patient's mouth by picking it up with the forefinger.

5. Place the loaded tray horizontally on a bracket table to minimize the flow of material out of the tray.

6. Have the dental assistant stand on the other side of the patient holding out a spatula with a small amount of alginate impression material taken from that remaining in the rubber bowl. Take it with your forefinger and place it in the patient's mouth (Fig. 3-3). This step is always used when making the maxillary impression and is occasionally used for some areas of the mandibular impression, as will be described. Have the assistant continue to supply additional material on the end of the spatula. When no more material is needed in the patient's mouth, proceed by seating the loaded tray. The assistant is responsible for cleaning the mixing bowl and spatula to prepare for additional impressions. The assistant also sets a timer for two minutes to mark the set of the material when using a Type II, normal-set alginate. Have him set the timer after you finish placing the impression material in the patient's mouth.

The technique of making the mandibular and maxillary impressions will now be described in more detail.

*L.D. Caulk Co., Milford, Del.

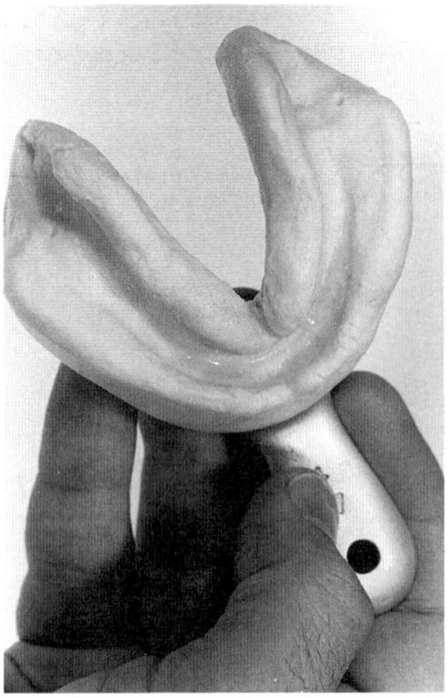

Fig. 3-4 Completed preliminary mandibular impression.

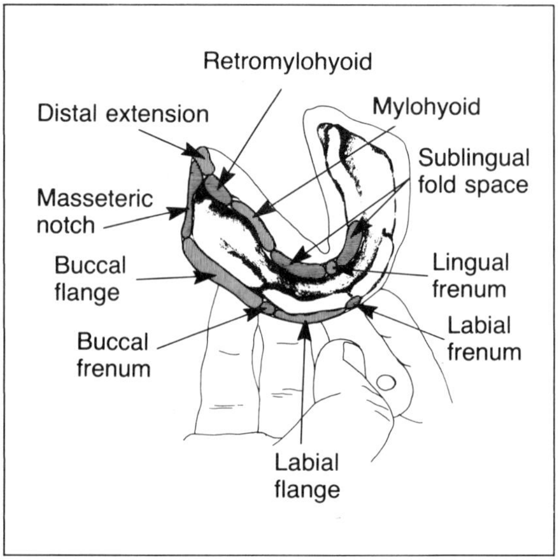

Fig. 3-5 The mandibular impression and the mandibular denture base are divided into ten areas for trimming the alginate, adjusting the custom tray, and molding the border.

The mandibular impression

Alginate material is not manually placed in the mouth because pooling of saliva in the mandibular arch often occurs too rapidly for successful use of the technique, and gravity allows these areas to fill in more completely than with a maxillary impression. If desired, alginate material can be wiped into areas that are undercut or were missed in previous attempts. Follow these steps:

1. Insert the loaded tray in the patient's mouth. Instruct the patient to lift his tongue up and out. While he is doing this, seat the impression tray posteriorly into the retromylohyoid area. This will allow a complete impression of the retromylohyoid area without the tongue blocking the flow of material. (It is a common error to get an impression of the base of the tongue in this area rather than of the entire retromylohyoid area because the patient did not lift his tongue.) Next, instruct the patient to relax his tongue in a protruded position. Continue to seat the tray anteriorly using the anterior flange of the stock tray as a guide. Express the material around the buccal and labial borders by lifting the cheeks and lip to mimic functional movements in these areas.
2. Lift the buccal fat pad over the distobuccal corner of the stock stray. As with the maxillary impression, whether or not you have properly captured the buccal and labial border extensions should be apparent. *Simply look while the impression is being made.*
3. Instruct the patient to close his mouth with his tongue in a relaxed forward position, stopping before contact is made between the maxilla and the tray. Hold the impression lightly in place for two minutes with no movement on your part or the patient's.
4. Remove the impression with one quick, controlled movement.
5. Inspect the impression for its acceptability (Fig. 3-4).

Trimming an alginate impression

Trimming an alginate impression is an art that must be learned and practiced. The objective is to create an impression that has the character and anatomic form of the patient and of the eventual finished denture base. Study the descriptions and illustrations on the following pages so that the desired shape and anatomic form become fixed in your mind and so that the objectives of trimming can be met.

Trimming the mandibular impression

Using a sharp scalpel blade, trim the impression to defined border landmarks to give it the character and anatomic form of the eventual finished denture base. This enables you to trim the custom impression tray in far less time, because the basic anatomic form has already been shaped in the alginate impression. The trimming of the mandibular impression is accomplished by dividing the impression into ten defined areas (Fig. 3-5).

Masseteric notch area

Trim this area at approximately a 45° angle to the buccal shelf. The angle formed in the impression itself between the buccal shelf and the masseteric notch area will usually be evident, and the trimming should follow it. Trim up to the distobuccal aspect of the retromolar pad.

Buccal flange and buccal frena

Trim the buccal flange at the area of the external oblique ridge. Then trim the buccal flange to be parallel to the crest of the residual ridge. Trim the buccal frenum bilaterally so as to notch and define its location. This will allow for visualization of the frena location on the cast and therefore on the custom resin impression tray that will be made.

Labial flange and labial frena

Trim this flange to 2 to 3 mm thick at its peripheral border. Also notch the labial frenum to define its location.

Retromylohyoid area and distal extension—retromolar pad

Trim the retromylohyoid curtain to drop straight down from the distal aspect of the retromolar pad. Trim the retromylohyoid area to approximately 3 mm thick to allow freedom of movement for the base of the tongue. Trim this area to include the most distal extension of the retromolar pad. The pterygomandibular raphe will often be evident and can be used as a landmark for the trimming of the posterior extension.

Mylohyoid area

Trim this area so as to remove any excess alginate material. Preserve the length of the impression material into the floor of the mouth so that material passes the mylohyoid ridge.

Sublingual fold space and labial frenum

Trim this area so as to remove any excess width of alginate material. Preserve the length of the impression material into the floor of the mouth. In this area, we are ultimately looking for a maximum extension in length and width of the denture border.

The maxillary impression

1. Remove alginate impression material from the spatula with your forefinger.

2. Ask the patient to partially close his mouth, and wipe material into both of the retrozygomatic areas opposite the tuberosities (Fig. 3-6). (If the patient's mouth is opened wide, the coronoid process will move forward and block material from entering.) Place alginate material in the remaining right and left labial and buccal vestibules. Place additional material to cover the palate. This will help minimize the entrapment of air in this area of the impression.

3. Pick up the impression tray and, from a position behind the patient, place the tray in the patient's mouth. (It is very difficult to manipulate the impression tray if you stand in front of the patient.) Use the anterior flange of the tray as a guide for the anterior-posterior positioning. Position the anterior metal flange of the tray so that it

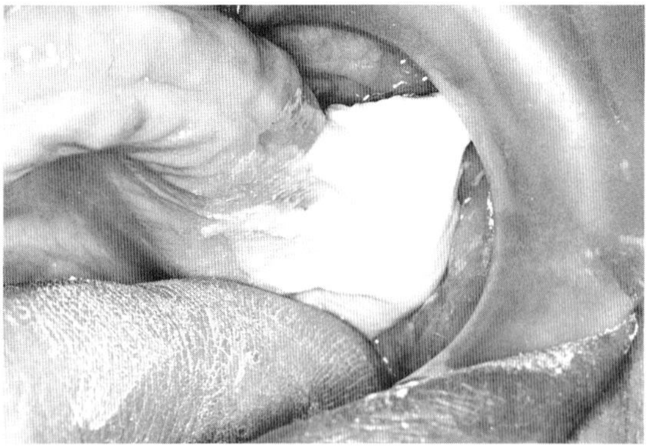

Fig. 3-6 Impression material is manually placed into both retrozygomatic areas. The remaining vestibular areas are also filled with alginate.

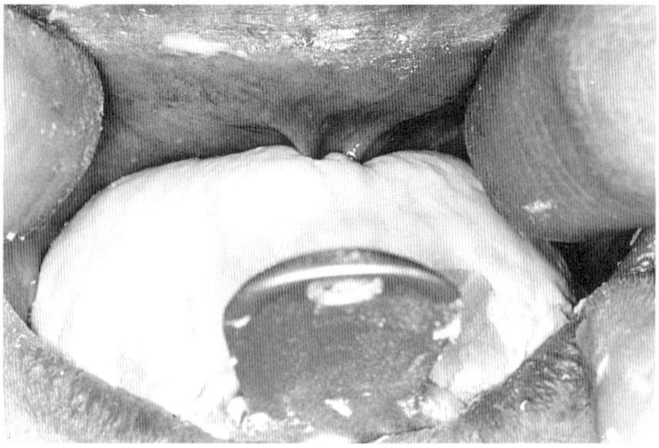

Fig. 3-7 Reflect the tissues of the lip and cheeks to visualize the adaptation of the alginate as the tray is being seated.

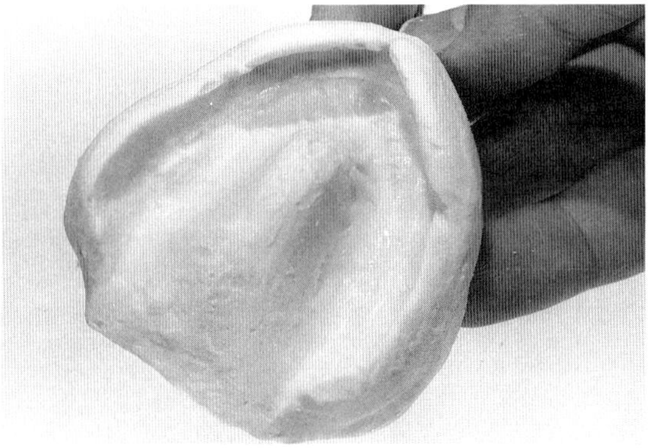

Fig. 3-8 Completed untrimmed preliminary maxillary impression.

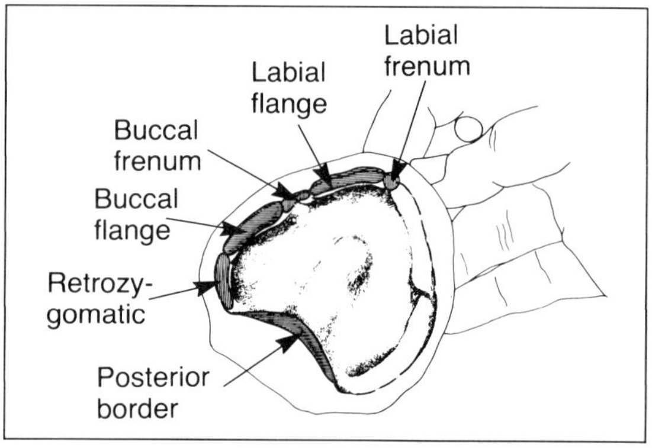

Fig. 3-9 The maxillary impression and the maxillary denture base are divided into six areas for trimming the alginate, adjusting the custom tray, and molding the border.

is in the proper border position. If the tray is not seated far enough posteriorly, the anterior alginate border will be posterior to the anterior labial flange of the tray. It therefore will not be accurately supported and, furthermore, the tuberosity will not be captured. Use the handle of the tray as a guide for the midline.

4. Exert bilateral pressure to express alginate material over the borders of the tray and form the peripheral roll in all areas. Keep in mind that you want the material that was manually placed into the mouth to coalesce with the tray-loaded material. Continue to seat the tray evenly while using your fingers to mold the cheeks and lip to form the periphery. Reflect the tissues of the lip and cheeks to visualize the adaptation of the alginate (Fig. 3-7). Make the necessary corrections while the alginate will still flow. Whether or not you have properly captured the peripheral borders of the labial or buccal flanges should be apparent.

5. Hold the impression lightly in place for two minutes with *absolutely no movement* by yourself or the patient. Do not clean the excess alginate material from your hands or write in the chart or get the next impression ready. Any movement by you or the patient will cause distortion of the impression.

6. Lift the lip away from the tray and remove

the impression with one quick, controlled movement.

7. Inspect the completed impression for acceptability (Fig. 3-8).

Trimming the maxillary impression

The objective of trimming the maxillary impression is the same as that of trimming the mandibular impression: to have it resemble the finished denture base. Again, trimming the height and the width of the periphery now saves much time in trimming the resin tray later. The custom resin tray that will be made from the preliminary impression will also be trimmed with the same anatomic areas in mind. Trim the impression as follows, defining border landmarks using a sharp scalpel blade. The impression is divided into six areas (Fig. 3-9).

Retrozygomatic and coronoid process areas

Trim these areas to conform to the approximate function of the coronoid process and to the height and width of the retrozygomatic area. Often the activity of the coronoid process is visible in the alginate impression. The coronoid process area is thinner in a denture base because of the action of the coronoid process and the temporal muscle against it; therefore, it must be trimmed in the impression. The retrozygomatic area is usually the thickest and highest area of the maxillary denture flanges. Do not reduce the height of the extension in this area.

Buccal flange and buccal frenum

Trim this area thicker than the labial flange, following the form developed in the alginate. Additional impression material can be removed from the buccal frena to define their location more clearly in the impression. This will allow for a more precise visualization of the frena location on the cast and, therefore, on the custom resin impression tray to be made.

Labial flange

Trim this area to approximately 2 to 3 mm thick. It should be thinner than the buccal flange. Remove additional impression material at the labial frenum to clearly define its location. This also will allow for visualization of the frenum location on the cast and on the custom resin impression tray.

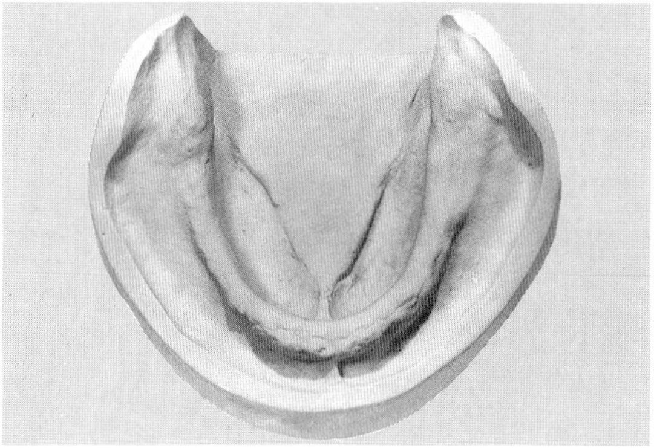

Fig. 3-10 A cast made from a preliminary maxillary alginate impression. Note the land area that frames the cast.

Posterior border area

Bilaterally trim the impression material through the hamular notches and the pterygomandibular raphe. The distance between the hamular notches is cut to the approximate area of the vibrating line, which is where the alginate begins to drop. Remove any excess impression material from the coronoid process to the hamular notch. Trim the distance between the hamular notches to define the posterior limit of the impression. The fovea palatinae, if impressed, cannot be used as a definite guideline for the posterior extension, because their position varies compared to the position of the vibrating line.[1] The vibrating line is the approximate area to which the most posterior border of the denture will ultimately extend. If in doubt leave additional alginate material in this area, as the final posterior border extensions will be determined during the secondary impression. In addition, the fovea are generally located anterior to the vibrating line. *The trimmed maxillary impression will resemble a completed denture base.*

Making accurate casts

The final step in completing the preliminary alginate impression is to form an accurate cast. Making accurate casts from preliminary alginate impressions does not occur by accident. Care must be exercised to retain the form that was captured in the impression. A cast can only be as good as the impression from which it is made. The cast must accurately reproduce the tissue detail of the denture-bearing areas as well as the height and width of the peripheral borders.

One of the most important goals is to pour the cast to achieve a land area that will frame the cast and preserve the height and width of the impressioned peripheral borders (Fig. 3-10).

References

1. Lye, T.L. The significance of the fovea palatini in complete denture prosthodontics. J. Prosthet. Dent. 33:504, 1975.

Make your preliminary alginate impression over and over again until it is right. The diagnostic cast that you make from it is as important as the final cast.

Allen Brewer
(Personal communication)

Chapter 4

Custom Impression Tray With Peripheral Relief

This chapter describes a technique for the fabrication of an impression tray that:

1. Is custom made
2. Is made from a cast that was poured from a preliminary alginate impression
3. Has relief space on the slopes of the ridges and on the peripheral border areas
4. Is a selective tissue placement tray
5. Can be made by manually adapting acrylic resin or by compression molding (flasking) acrylic resin

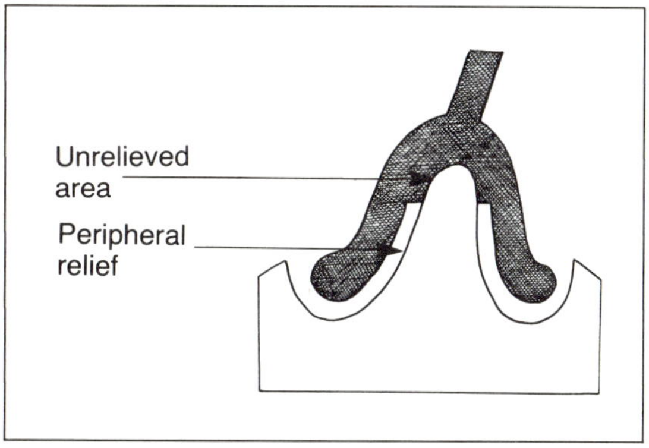

Fig. 4-1a Maxillary custom impression tray with peripheral relief. The slopes of the ridges are relieved away from the cast, whereas the ridge crest areas are closely adapted to the cast.

Philosophy of the custom impression tray with peripheral relief

A specially designed custom tray with peripheral relief spaces is fabricated (Figs. 4-1a and b). While the preliminary alginate impression will record the attached mucosa of the ridge crest with less tissue placement, compound impression material records the movable tissues on the slopes of the ridges and peripheral sulcus areas with additional placement and pressure. The slopes of the ridges are considered primary supporting areas, and the impression techniques to be described selectively load these tissues. Compound impression material can be added to or taken away from the impression to complete it while achieving the maximum in sta-

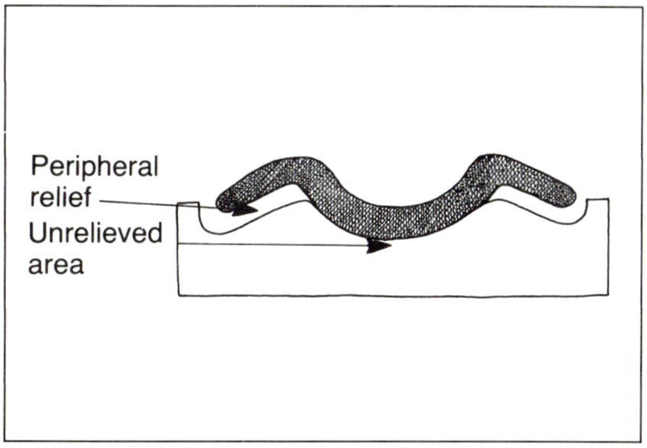

Fig. 4-1b Mandibular custom impression tray with peripheral relief.

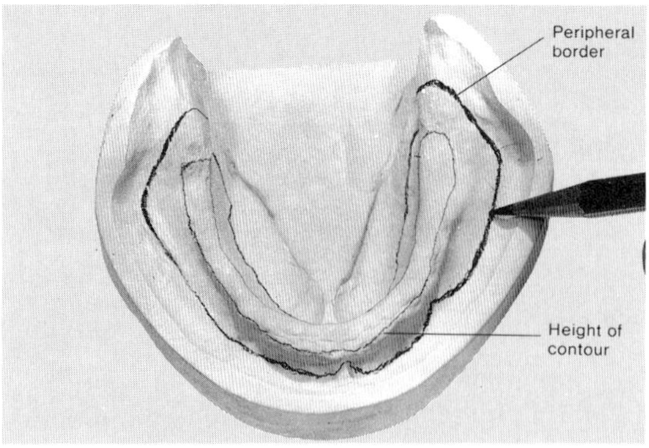

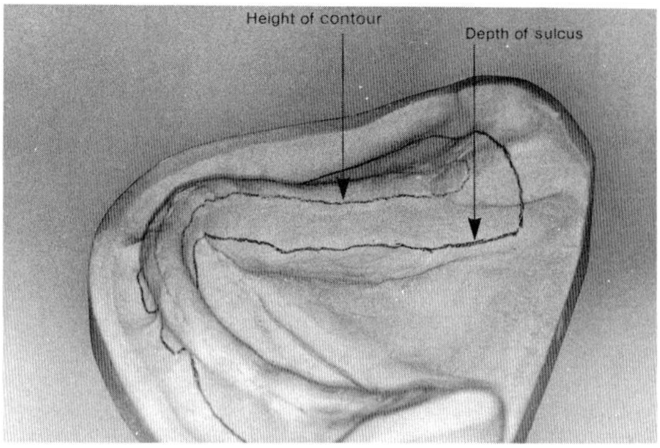

Figs. 4-2a and b The depth of the sulcus and the height of the contour of the ridge are marked in pencil. The area between these two lines is where the wax relief will be placed.

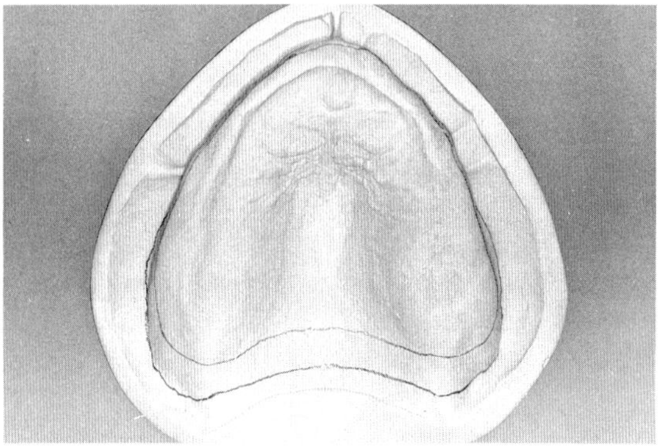

Fig. 4-2c The posterior palatal seal areas are treated in a similar manner.

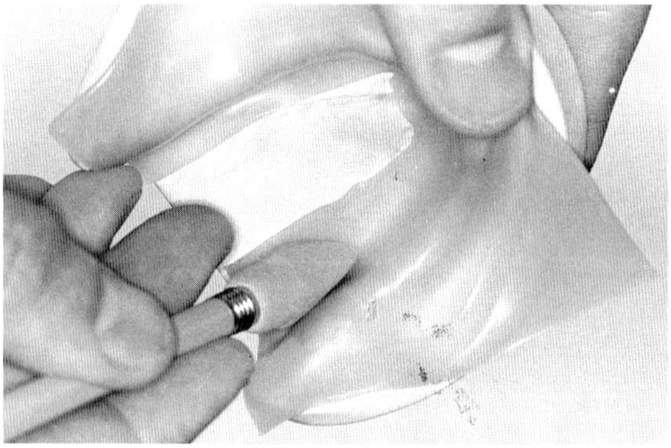

Fig. 4-3 One layer of warmed wax is adapted to the entire cast.

bility and retention. The unrelieved portion of the tray is the final impression for that area; therefore, no impression material is placed over it. The unrelieved portion of the tray supports the tray to its fullest seating, providing rest and stability during the border molding procedures. This border-molded tray becomes the final impression without the need to add a "wash" impression inside of it.

The custom impression tray with peripheral relief can be made with or without compression-molded acrylic resin. Both techniques (compression molded and manually adapted) will be described. The compression-molded tray is made by first waxing up the tray and flasking it as you would a finished denture. The manually adapted tray is made without flasking; autopolymerizing acrylic resin is manually adapted to a specially prepared cast. The wax relief space is made in the same manner regardless of which technique is used.

The wax relief

The purpose of this relief is to provide space between the tissue and the tray. The controlled space will allow an even thickness of compound to be placed during border molding. The unrelieved acrylic resin surfaces will allow for accurate repositioning of the tray in the mouth during border molding. Follow these steps:

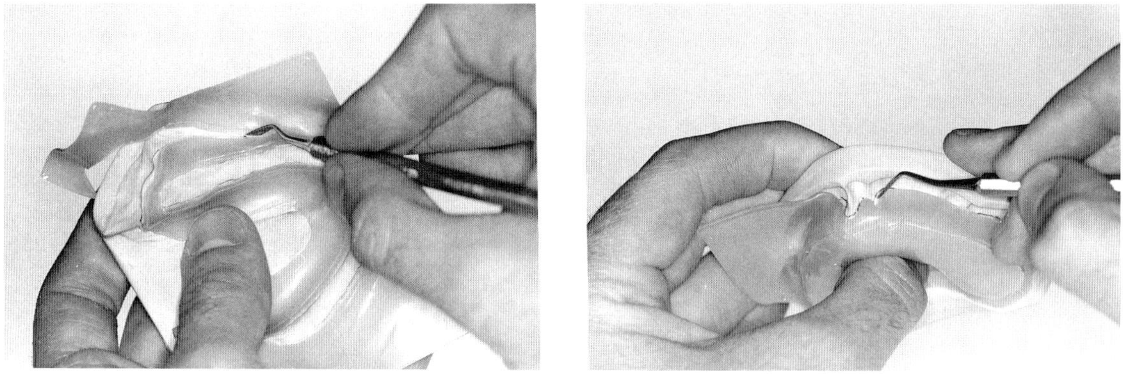

Figs. 4-4a and b The wax is cut at right angles to the pencilled lines with a sharp instrument.

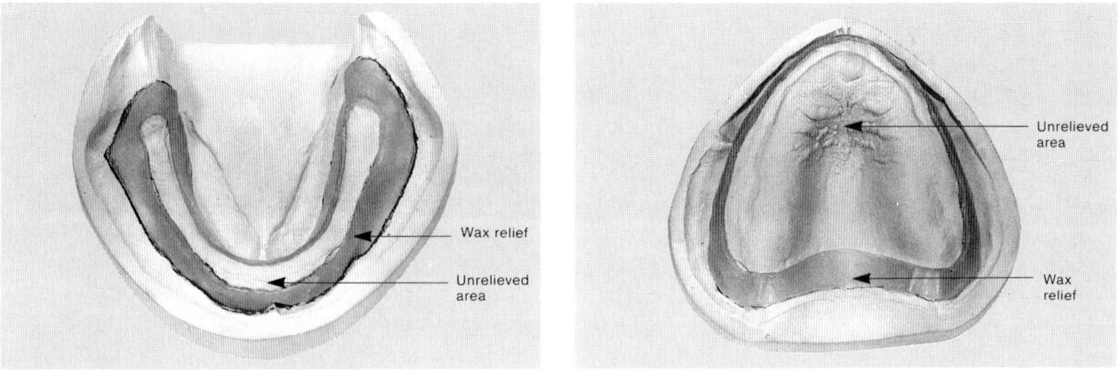

Figs. 4-5a and b The wax occupies the space between the two pencilled lines.

1. Outline in pencil on the cast the circumference of the depth of the sulcus. Draw another line around the circumference of the height of contour of the denture-bearing area (Figs. 4-2a to c). This results in two separate, continuous lines. The area between these two lines is to be the area of wax relief.

2. Create the wax relief by adapting one layer of warmed 1 mm-thick wax (Thin-Ex Wax*) to the entire cast (Fig. 4-3). Use a pencil eraser tip to adapt the wax.

*Modern Materials Mfg. Co., St. Louis, Mo.

3. Use a sharp blade to cut the wax along and at right angles to the pencilled lines (Figs. 4-4a and b). It is important that a clean, defined butt joint be created. After the wax has been cut, remove and discard the excess wax above the ridge crest, leaving only the wax relief—the wax located around the periphery of the cast between the pencilled lines (Figs. 4-5a and b). It is important not to extend the relief wax to fill up the peripheral border of the cast because it will cover the anatomic landmarks essential to the design of the tray. This detail will help you to properly trim the tray after it is made and before the patient visit.

4. Remove the wax relief from the cast and set it aside for later use.

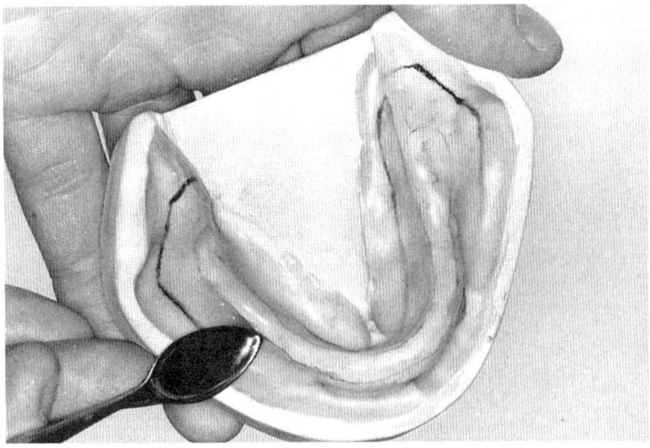

Fig. 4-6 Melt fluid baseplate wax over the entire cast.

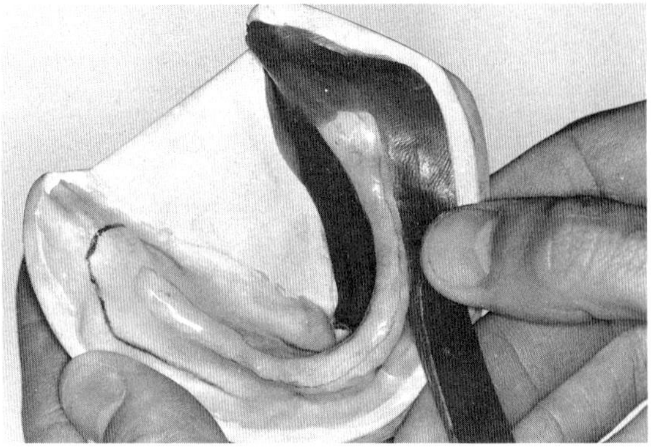

Figs. 4-7a and b Utility wax is adapted around the periphery up to the height of contour of the cast at the pencilled line.

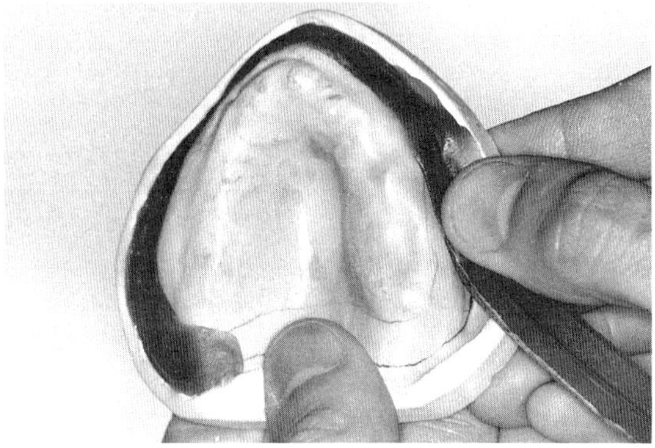

Fig. 4-7b

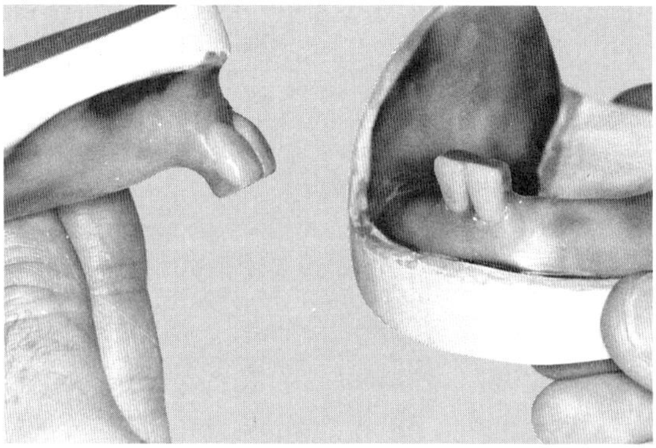

Fig. 4-8 The handle is waxed and positioned to simulate the eventual position of the maxillary and mandibular teeth. The teeth are in position here only to dramatize the importance of handle placement and size.

Compression-molded acrylic resin impression tray

The wax-up for the custom tray

1. Melt a small quantity of baseplate wax over the entire dry cast to ensure wax adaptation and adherence for the tray wax-up (Fig. 4-6).

2. Adapt utility wax strips around the periphery up to the height of contour of the cast at the pencilled lines (Figs. 4-7a and b). The utility wax should fill the entire width of the sulcus and provide the needed thickness to the tray.

3. Place a sheet of baseplate wax over the entire cast and over the utility wax strips. Trim and contour the wax to the art border of the cast.

4. Mold a wax handle onto the waxed-up tray. Place the handle slightly anterior to the ridge to simulate the position of the anterior teeth (Fig. 4-8). The handle should be large enough for ease of manipulation in and out of the mouth.

5. Flask the cast in plaster using two pours. First pour the lower half (Fig. 4-9). When this sets, place a thin layer of separating medium (petroleum jelly or soap) on the exposed plaster. Then pour the upper half of the flask. After the plaster is set, place the flask in boiling water. Allow the wax to soften for about four minutes. Open the flask. Lift off the warmed waxed-up tray and discard. Thoroughly

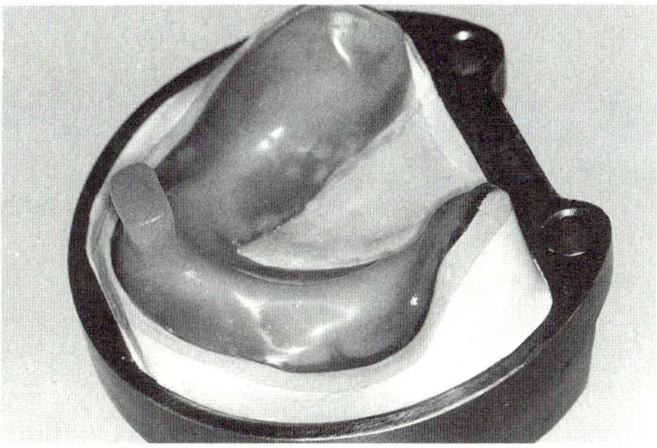

Fig. 4-9 The waxed-up cast is flasked in a conventional manner using plaster.

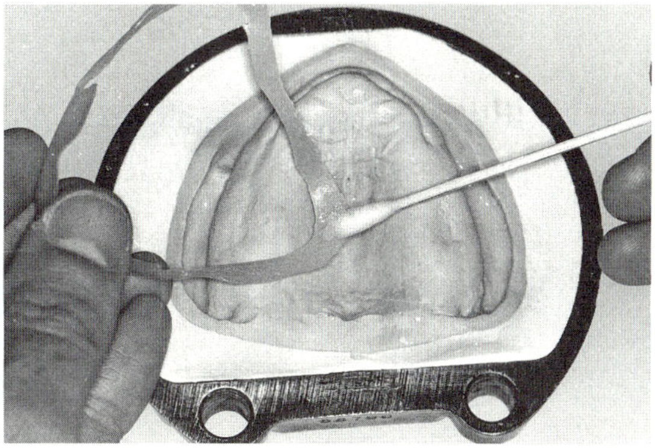

Fig. 4-10a Household cement is applied to the undersurface of the wax.

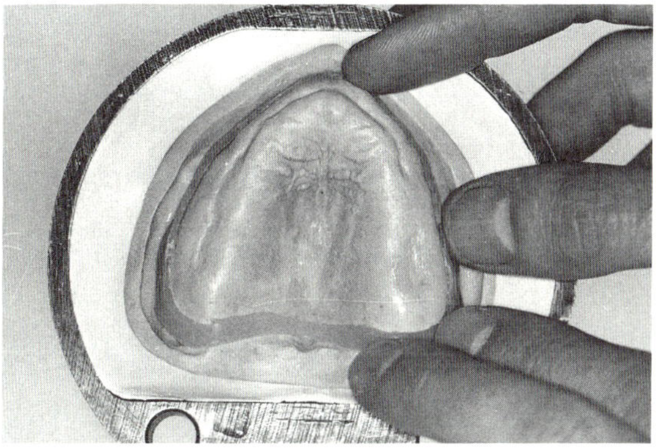

Fig. 4-10b The wax relief is glued to the cast surface.

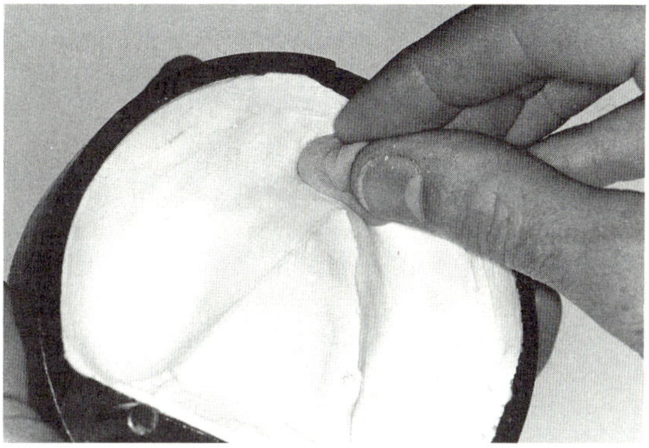

Fig. 4-11 Additional acrylic resin is placed in the handle hole during packing.

flush the remaining wax away with detergent and three rinses of clean, boiling water. Allow the cast to cool and dry.

Processing the custom tray

1. Glue the previously made wax relief to the cast with a household cement (Duco Cement*) (Figs. 4-10a and b). The cement ensures that the wax will stay in place during packing and curing.
2. Paint one layer of tinfoil substitute onto all stone surfaces and allow it to dry.

*Dupont Co., Wilmington, Del.

3. Mix an autopolymerizing acrylic resin according to the manufacturer's directions. Adapt the resin to the flask while the resin is in its doughy stage. Place some resin in the handle hole to ensure its complete packing (Fig. 4-11). Close the flask and tighten it securely using a flask press. Allow the resin to bench set for 45 minutes.
4. Remove the flask from the press and separate the stone from the flask by using a flask ejector.*
5. Place the entire plaster unit under hot running tap water for approximately five minutes. This will soften the wax relief, allowing the two stone parts and the resin tray to separate easily.

*Teledyne Dental—Hanau Div., Buffalo, N.Y.

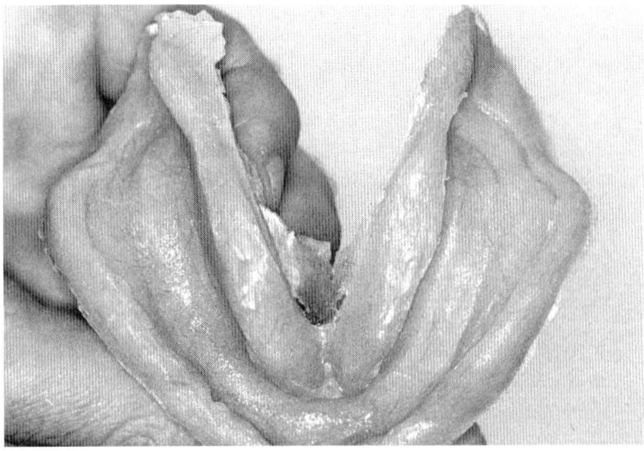

Fig. 4-12 The custom tray after deflasking.

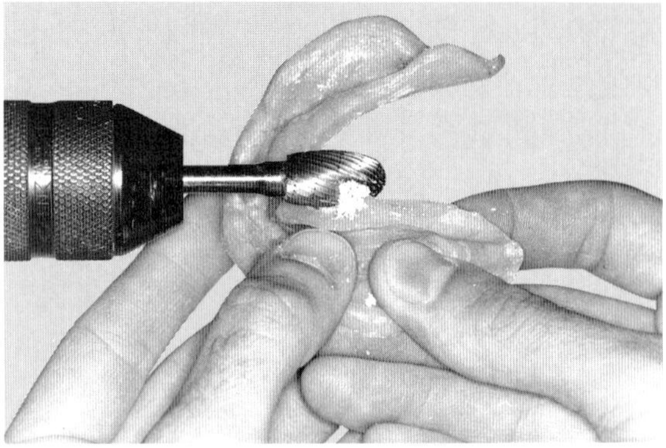

Fig. 4-13 Arbor bands and large carbide burs in a lathe make the gross trimming easier and more efficient.

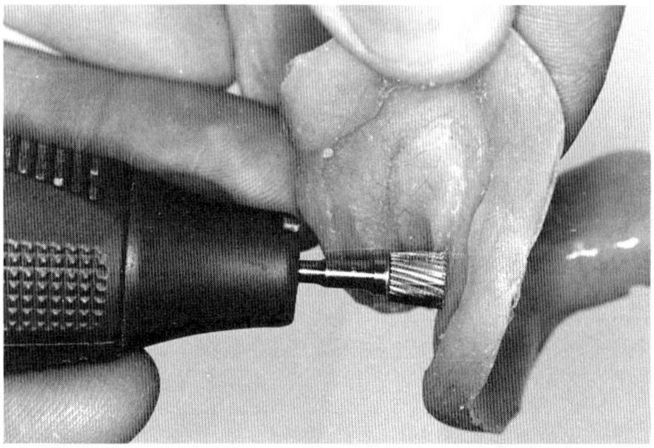

Fig. 4-14 The peripheral borders of the custom tray are relieved so that the tray is level with the space created by the wax relief.

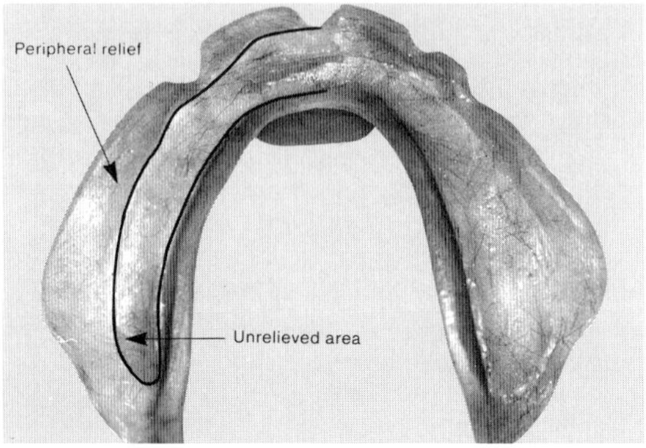

Fig. 4-15a The mandibular impression tray has been made but not yet adjusted for the patient's mouth.

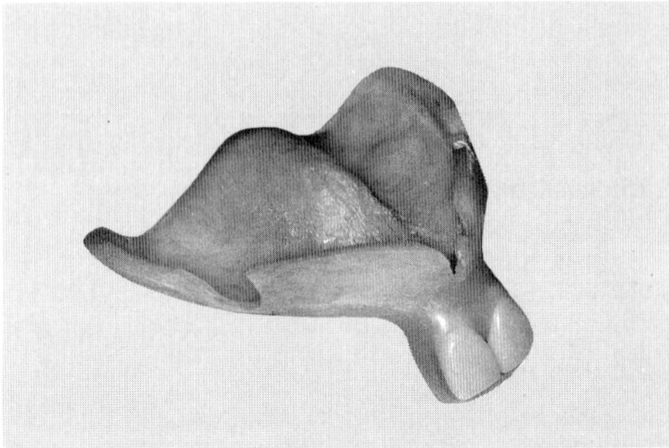

Fig. 4-15b The completed maxillary impression tray has teeth attached to dramatize tray handle position.

6. Retrieve the resin tray and clean away any adherent wax (Fig. 4-12). Redefine the butt joint in the acrylic resin at the height of contour by using an inverted cone laboratory carbide bur. The butt joint was originally created by the wax relief.

7. Trim the excess flash remaining on the tray using arbor bands and carbide burs (Fig. 4-13). Use the anatomical landmarks incorporated into the resin tray by trimming the alginate impression as described in chapter 3 as guidelines for trimming the tray. Trim the tray area by area, in the manner previously described for trimming the alginate impression. The outline of the trimmed tray should resemble a completed denture base. While trimming the borders, reduce the added thickness of resin at the depth of the sulcus to be flush with the spaced area created by the wax relief. There is now one thickness of relieved area from the height of contour to the land area. This relief measures approximately 1 mm (Fig. 4-14).

8. The processed custom tray has been completed but not yet adjusted for the patient (Figs. 4-15a and b). The final adjustments of the tray are accomplished with the patient prior to making the secondary impression. The technique for adjusting the maxillary and mandibular trays is detailed in chapters 6 and 7.

Manually adapted acrylic resin impression tray

1. Glue the wax relief to the cast with an epoxy cement. The cement ensures that the wax will stay in place while the acrylic resin is added.

2. Paint one layer of tinfoil substitute onto the cast and allow it to dry.

3. Sprinkle autopolymerizing repair resin (polymer) powder onto the cast and saturate it with the monomer liquid (Fig. 4-16). Continue to apply material until the repair resin fills the entire unrelieved area of the cast up to and slightly over the wax butt joint.

4. Make a separate mix of autocuring impression tray acrylic resin, form the resin into a roll, and fill the peripheral border areas with resin (Fig. 4-17).

5. Adapt additional acrylic resin that has been flattened into an approximately 2-mm-thick sheet over the repair acrylic resin, wax spacer, and peripheral acrylic resin (Figs. 4-18a and b). Use acrylic resin to wax-up the tray with the same dimensions and thicknesses as with the flasking technique.

6. Use additional acrylic resin to form and add a handle to the tray.

7. Cure the impression tray in a pressure pot immersed in warm water for 20 minutes at 30 psi to reduce porosity in the acrylic resin.

8. Place the impression tray in a bowl of warm water to heat the peripheral relief wax. This will soften the wax and make it easier to remove the impression tray from the cast. Remove the impression tray.

9. To trim and finish the manually adapted tray, follow steps 6 to 8 of the instructions for trimming and finishing the compression-molded tray (Figs. 4-19a and b).

Alternative impression tray technique (light cured method)

1. Glue the wax relief to the cast with an epoxy cement. The cement ensures that the wax will stay in place while the acrylic resin is added.

2. Paint one thin coat of Model Release Agent* onto the cast.

3. Adapt Triad* VLC denture base material over the ridgecrest and palate, being careful to not trap air while placing the material. Adapt from center out after coating fingers with Air Barrier Coating* liquid, being careful to not contact areas where second layer of material would be added.

4. Adapt a second layer of Triad VLC denture base material over the ridge of the mandibular cast and periphery if thin in order to provide rigidity to the tray. Trim the excess material with a knife.

*Dentsply International, Inc., York, Pa.

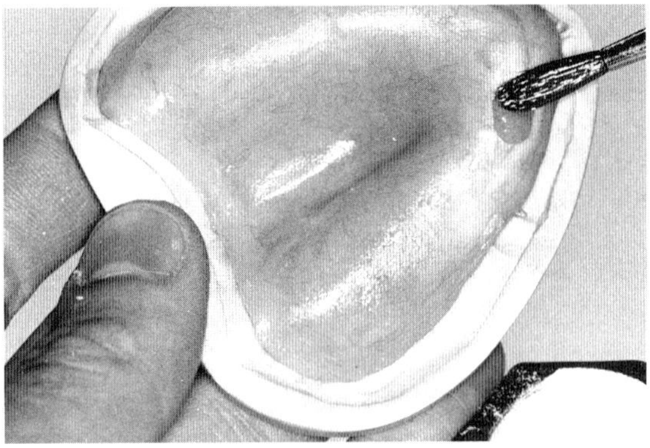

Fig. 4-16 Autopolymerizing repair resin is used to fill the unrelieved portion of the cast. This area is built up to be level with the wax relief.

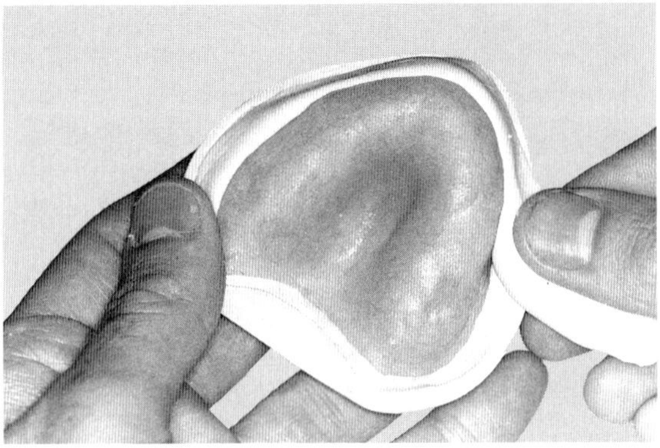

Fig. 4-17 The peripheral border areas are filled with impression tray acrylic resin.

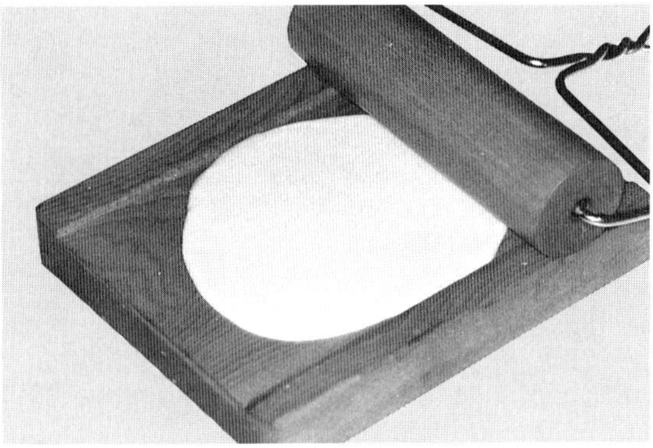

Fig. 4-18a Additional impression tray acrylic resin is flattened.

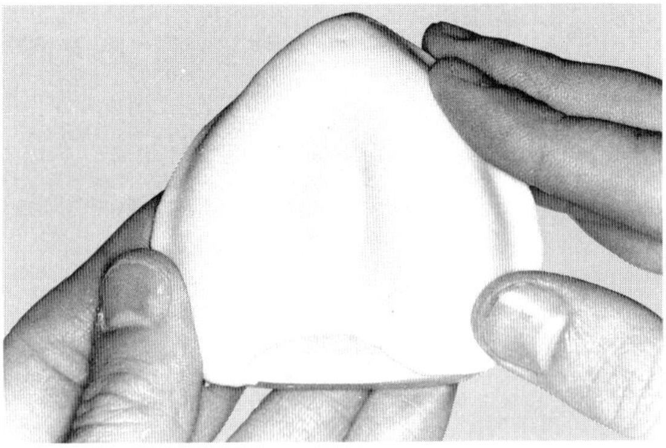

Fig. 4-18b The additional resin is adapted over the entire cast.

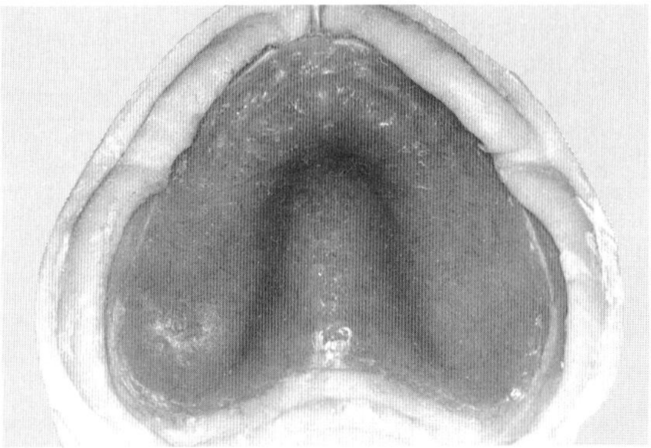

Fig. 4-19a Untrimmed maxillary impression tray.

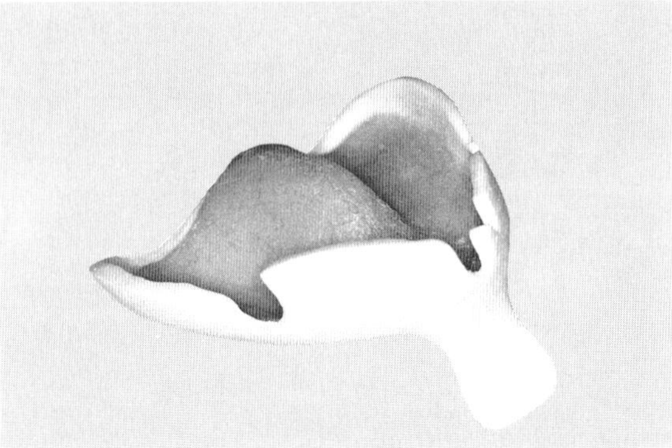

Fig. 4-19b Impression tray completed and ready for try-in.

5. Take a small amount of visible light cured material and form a handle. Use a portable light curing unit (Prisma*) to provide a preliminary cure to the handle, in order to prevent slumping.

*Dentsply International, Inc., York, Pa.

6. Cure the adapted tray in the Triad light curing unit (with turn table) for eight to ten minutes.

7. The impression tray can be *carefully* removed by placing it in hot water for two to three minutes as previously described; then it is trimmed and finished as for the compression-molded tray.

If the dentist knows his patient and if he understands what he wants to capture and create, then perhaps any of several techniques and materials will work. You can make an impression out of most any material if you know what you are doing. All good impressions look alike because we all are the same species of animal with the same anatomy.

Allen Brewer
(Personal communication)

Chapter 5

Mandibular Final Impression

The mandibular final impression procedure is accomplished by using the custom tray with the peripheral relief. This tray, as described in chapter 4, has an unrelieved area on the crest of the ridge and a relieved area on the slopes of the ridge and the peripheral border (see Figs. 4-1a and 4-15a). The unrelieved area of the tray is intimately adapted to the tissues of the crest of the ridge. Because no impression material is added to this area, it provides a stable and controlled position to which the tray is repeatedly returned while the final border molding is being accomplished. Therefore, the borders can be changed by trial and error (the compound can be added and removed) until the desired completed impression is obtained. The relieved area of the tray is the space in which the impression compound is added. Making an impression tray in this manner enables the dentist to produce a selective tissue placement impression *without* the use of a wash impression material such as zinc oxide–eugenol or rubber base within the border-molded tray.

Border molding of the final impression will be described in this chapter. The hard and soft tissues that mold the compound in each peripheral border area, the techniques that dentist and patient can use to activate the tissues for each border area, and the muscular or tissue movement that each of these techniques accomplishes will be discussed.

The purpose of border molding the mandibular denture is to create a peripheral seal in each extension area. The concept of an overall peripheral seal for a maxillary denture is commonly spoken of and easily understood. Mandibular denture base extensions should be thought of in exactly the same way.

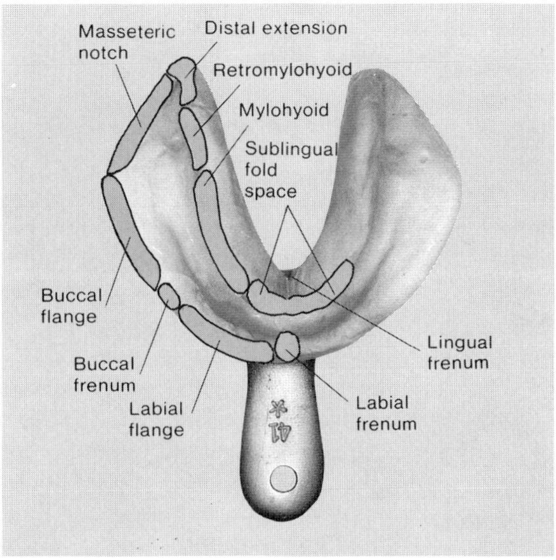

Fig. 5-1 The mandibular denture base is divided into ten anatomic areas. The preliminary alginate impression was trimmed using these areas for reference. Likewise, the final impression is completed using the same areas for reference.

Adjusting the custom tray to ten anatomic areas

The custom tray is trimmed and adjusted using the guidelines presented for the ten anatomic areas involved in trimming the preliminary alginate

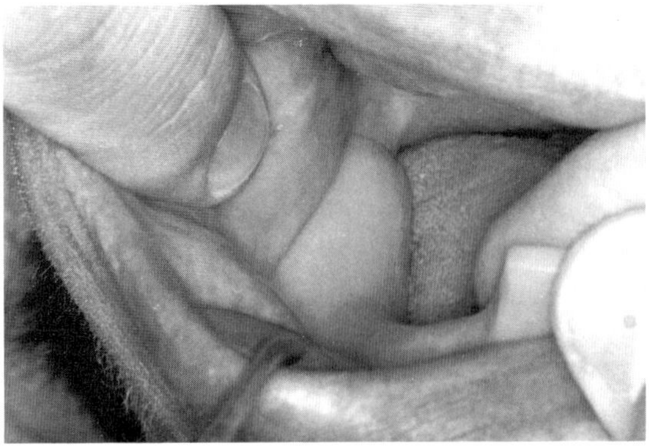

Fig. 5-2 The buccal fat pad assumes an undistorted position overlying the masseteric notch region of the denture base.

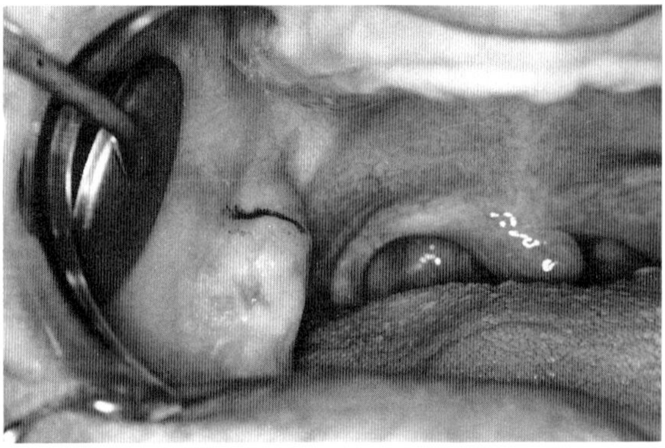

Fig. 5-3 A disposable marker is used to visually locate the distal extent of the retromolar pad.

impression (Fig. 5-1). The objectives of adjusting the impression tray at this time are *(1)* to trim the peripheral borders 2 to 3 mm short of the ultimate denture borders, and *(2)* to make an impression tray that has the appearance of the completed impression. The amount of retention and stability that the final mandibular impression will have is directly related to the quality and fit of the impression tray.

Trimming the impression tray

The first step in trimming is to place the impression tray in the patient's mouth and examine it. It is then adjusted where indicated, area by area, as follows.

Masseteric notch and distal extension areas

Trim the masseteric notch area to form an appropriate angle to the buccal shelf. The degree of the angle that is formed between the two areas varies from patient to patient but often approximates 45°. The masseteric notch region of the denture base is angled from the buccal shelf principally because of the action of the masseter muscle and the bony anatomy of the region. As the masseter muscle contracts, it pulls medially and therefore molds the impression material in that direction. The distobuccal corner between the masseteric notch and the buccal flange should be rounded, and the masseteric notch should be slightly concave. It should not displace the buccal fat pad but allow the pad to assume an undistorted position overlying the masseteric notch of the tray (Fig. 5-2).

The distal extension area of the impression tray is trimmed by looking at a combination of two factors, one anatomic and the other functional:

Anatomic factor. Adjust the tray to cover the retromolar pad. This is done by visually locating the retromolar pad and marking its distal extent with a disposable marker (Dr. Thompson's Color Transfer Applicators*) (Fig. 5-3).

Functional factor. Instruct the patient to open wide. This causes the pterygomandibular raphe to stretch. The raphe often attaches distal to the retromolar pad region. During border molding, the raphe is sometimes registered in the impression material. The distal extension area of the tray should just contact the pterygomandibular raphe when the mouth is partially closed.

Buccal flange and buccal frenum

Adjust the buccal flange to a line parallel to the ridge crest and 2 to 3 mm short of the external oblique ridge. Check this by palpating the external

*Great Plains Dental Products Co., Kingman, Kan.

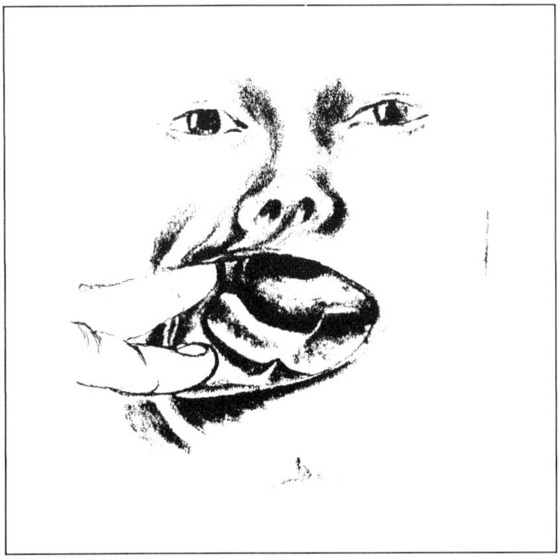

Fig. 5-4a The buccal flange is adjusted to be 2 to 3 mm short of the external oblique ridge; this is checked intraorally by using the ball of the index finger.

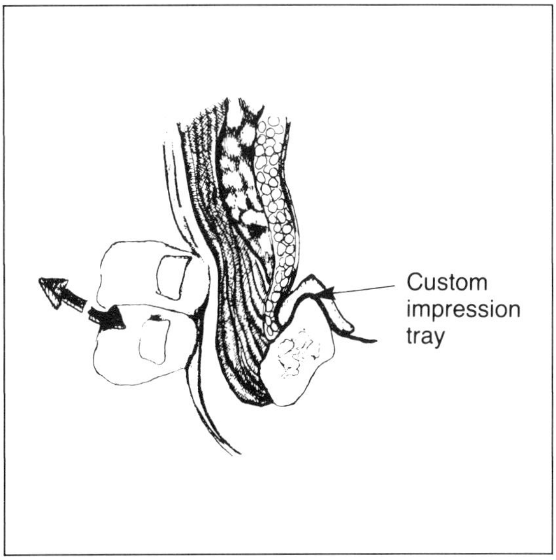

Fig. 5-4b The outer surface of the cheek is palpated to feel any overextension.

oblique ridge and the edge of the tray intraorally using the ball of the index finger (Fig. 5-4a). You should feel the external oblique ridge and the tray border simultaneously. Also use extraoral palpation of the cheek to ensure that the tray is not overextended in this region (Fig. 5-4b). As is true with the masseteric notch area, the tissues of the cheek should drape upon the outer surface of the impression tray in this region. Adjust the buccal frena areas until there is no interference when the frena are manually manipulated within the range of normal function (Fig. 5-5).

Labial flange and labial frenum

Adjust the labial flange of the tray until there is no muscle or tissue interference and until the tray is about 2 mm short of the tissue flexion line when the lip is gently reflected horizontally. Pulling the lip up or down can provide a false indication of the appropriate position of the vestibule in relation to the denture border. Palpate the lip extraorally to feel for overextensions. Adjust the labial frenum until there is no interference when the frenum is manually manipulated in any functional direction.

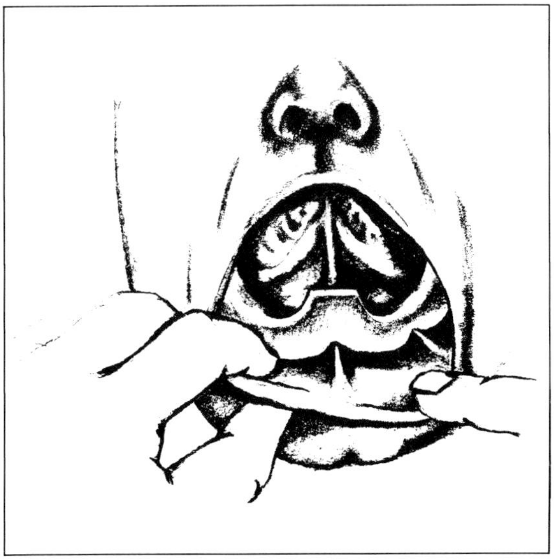

Fig. 5-5 The labial and buccal frenum areas of the tray are adjusted so that the lip and cheek can be moved within the range of normal function without interference.

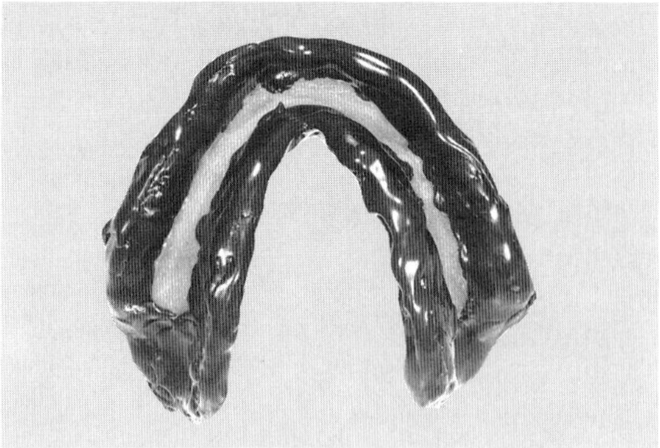

Fig. 5-6 All the relieved areas of the custom tray are generously filled with compound.

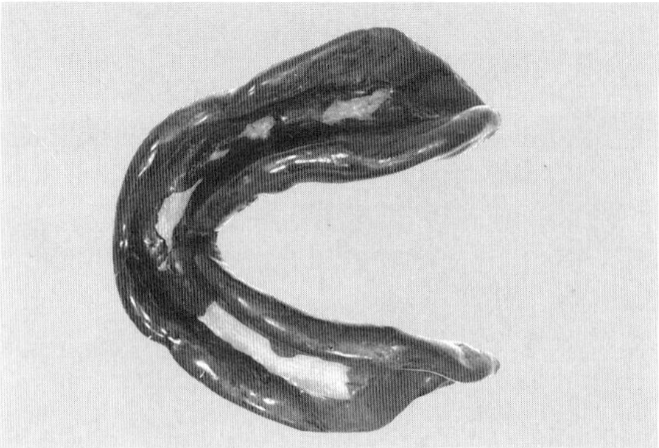

Fig. 5-7 Excess compound has flowed over the butt joint onto the unrelieved portion of the tray.

Retromylohyoid and mylohyoid areas

Instruct the patient to protrude his tongue as far as possible while you hold the tray in position. Adjust the retromylohyoid area until the dislodging forces seem to be slightly less in this area than in the mylohyoid region. This is determined by placing your index finger into these regions to feel the tension on the floor of the mouth. The retromylohyoid area should be thin and contoured to allow for free tongue movement. Instruct the patient to put his tongue into the opposite vestibule as if to clear out food from the area, a function he will have to perform during every meal. The outer surface of the tray in both areas should be concave to allow the tongue at rest to stabilize the tray during the impression procedure. Further trimming of the lingual border of the tray may be necessary after the compound has been added during border-molding procedures. Overextended areas of the tray usually show through the compound in this region.

Sublingual fold space and lingual frenum

Instruct the patient to gently place the tip of his tongue against the tray handle, which represents the position of the incisal edges of the anterior teeth. Adjust the tray until it is about 1 mm from the floor of the mouth when the tongue is in this position. View the lingual frenum area with a mirror while having the patient protrude his tongue directly forward and side to side. Adjust the tray to allow adequate freedom for tongue movement.

Making the mandibular final impression

Impression compound is now added to the relieved areas and to the periphery of the custom tray. The impression is perfected in two stages: *(1)* the initial adaptation of the compound and *(2)* the border molding to completion of the final impression. The most distolingual border of the denture area is called the *retromylohyoid curtain*. The tray in this area should approximate a right angle with the floor of the mouth.

Initial adaptation of the compound

1. Use the flame from a Bunsen burner to soften the end of a stick of impression compound. Generously fill all the relieved areas of the tray up to the butt joint with compound (Fig. 5-6). Place additional compound around the entire periphery.
2. Use the flame from an alcohol torch to soften the compound on the tray, and dip the tray in a water bath at the working temperature of the compound to temper and evenly soften the compound.
3. Place the tray in the patient's mouth and seat it slowly, allowing the compound to flow (Fig.

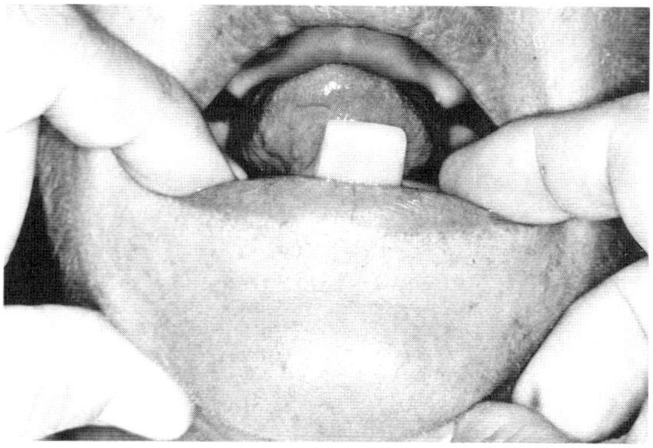

Fig. 5-8a The patient is instructed to raise his tongue above the handle of the tray and to protrude it straight out of his mouth.

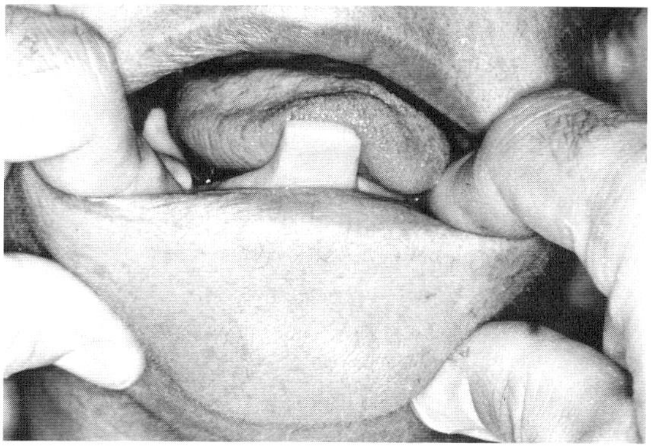

Fig. 5-8b The patient is instructed to move his tongue to each corner of the mouth.

5-7). Repeat steps 1, 2, and 3 until the compound has flowed over the entire butt joint and filled all areas of the relieved portion of the tray. If voids exist, add more compound. If compound does not flow over all areas of the butt joint, you cannot be sure that enough compound was added, so additional compound should be placed in these areas. This may involve several trial insertions.

4. Remove the tray from the mouth and chill it in ice water. Scrape the excess compound back to the butt joint using a small vulcanite scraper, being careful not to mar the acrylic resin tray.

5. Reheat the compound and repeat steps 3 and 4 until no compound covers the unrelieved portion of the tray.

Border molding and completing the impression

Before border molding by area, reheat the compound in the water bath and return it to the mouth. Hold it down firmly. Tell the patient to raise his tongue above the handle of the tray, protrude it straight out of his mouth, to both corners, then back to its normal position while you hold the tray in position (Figs. 5-8a and b).

Check for overextensions of the retromylohyoid and mylohyoid areas. If the tray shows through in either of these areas, trim the tray back and add more compound. Repeat this until the tray acrylic resin is not exposed. The amount of compound in the sublingual fold space limits the amount of protrusion that the tongue can accomplish. The length of the impression tray in this area prevents the overshortening of the lingual flange in the retromylohyoid and mylohyoid areas by limiting the tongue's movement.

Masseteric notch and distal extension areas

Dry the compound and flame heat the masseteric notch and distal extension areas (Table 5-1) bilaterally.

Temper and place the impression in the mouth and hold the tray in position bilaterally. Instruct the patient to open wide and then to close on the tray handle or against the resisting force of your fingers. Opening wide activates the muscles of the pterygomandibular raphe as it causes the raphe to stretch. This stretching impresses the raphe against the compound and defines the most distal extension of the impression. It is important to mold this area to cover the retromolar pad and to end the impression on the displaceable tissue distal to it. This allows the denture base to cover the maximum amount of bearing area and to be sealed on displaceable tissue. Instructing the patient to close against your fingers on the tray handle causes the masseter muscle to contract and push against the medially situated buccinator muscle and adjacent soft tissues and softened compound (Figs. 5-9a and b).

Reheat the compound in the masseteric notch area on one side and insert the tray. Hold the tray

Table 5-1 Masseteric notch and distal extension areas

Anatomic region	Tissues that influence extension	How to activate	What activation accomplishes
Masseteric notch	Masseter muscle Buccinator muscle Buccal fat pad	Instruct patient to close down on your fingers and the tray handle	Masseter muscle contracts against buccinator muscle
		Manually manipulate the buccal fat pad by drawing the cheek up to bring excess compound onto the tray	Buccal fat pad is elevated onto outer peripheral border to help seal and stabilize denture
Distal extension area	Pterygomandibular raphe Retromolar pad	Have patient open his mouth wide	Pterygomandibular raphe stretches, capturing the raphe and defining the most distal extension of the impression
			Denture base covers the maximum amount of bearing area and is sealed on displaceable tissue

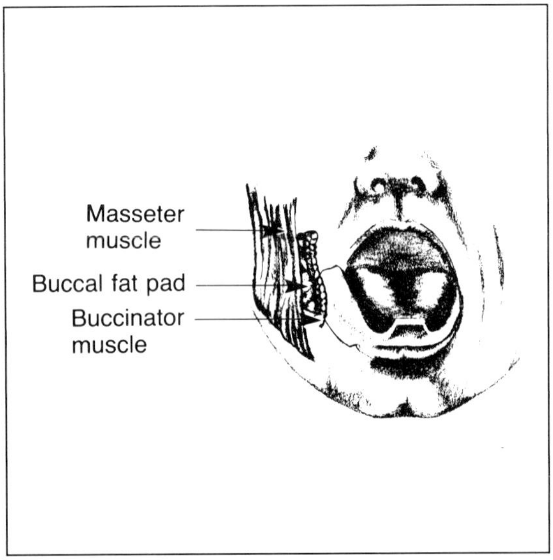

Fig. 5-9a The tissues that influence the extension of the denture base in the masseteric notch region are shown.

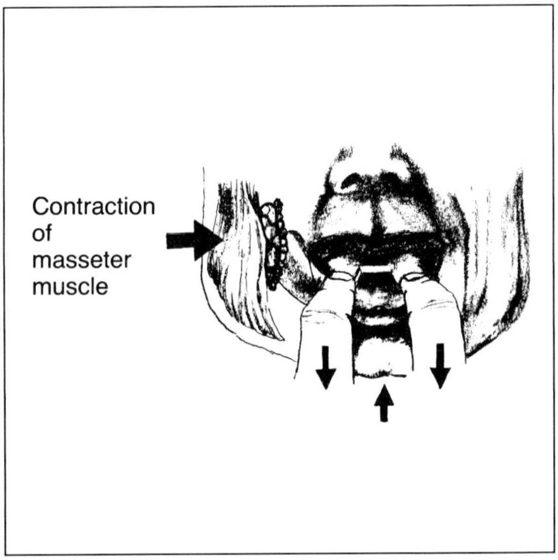

Fig. 5-9b The masseter muscle is activated by instructing the patient to close against your resisting force *(arrows)*. This activity causes the masseter muscle to contract inward with force against the buccinator muscle and therefore against the impression material.

securely with one hand while the other hand draws the cheek up and brings excess compound onto the outer tray surface (Fig. 5-10). This action manually manipulates the buccal fat pad onto and over the outer border. This permits the fat pad tissues to rest upon the outer surface of the denture border, which helps stabilize and seal the denture. Repeat the procedure for the other side. Chill and dry the compound.

Buccal flange and buccal frenum areas

Flame heat the buccal flange area (Table 5-2) bilaterally. Temper and place it in the mouth.

Hold the tray in position with one hand. Mold by massaging the cheek in an anterior-posterior direction using moderate manual pressure against the compound (Fig. 5-11). This moves the fibers of the buccinator muscle and the tissues of the cheek in the direction of the functional action of the buccinator muscle. Look at the flange extension in the mouth to see that the cheek contour is not disturbed and that the tissues of the cheek rest unstrained upon the outer surface of the impression tray. Feel the border of the flange with the ball of the index finger to check for overextension. The outer border of this flange is usually parallel to the crest of the ridge. The external oblique ridge is also used as a landmark; the denture border should extend up to but not beyond it. Palpate the cheek externally to check for overextension. It is also important to look at the patient's facial form for esthetic purposes to determine if the area is overextended.

Flame heat the buccal frena area on one side. Temper and place it in the mouth holding the tray in position with one hand. With the other hand, elevate the frenum into the compound and then mold the cheek in an anterior-posterior direction. The anterior-posterior movement allows freedom of the frena while maintaining peripheral contact. Repeat for the opposite side.

Labial flange and labial frenum

Flame heat the labial flange (Table 5-3). Temper and place it in the mouth holding the tray in position with one hand.

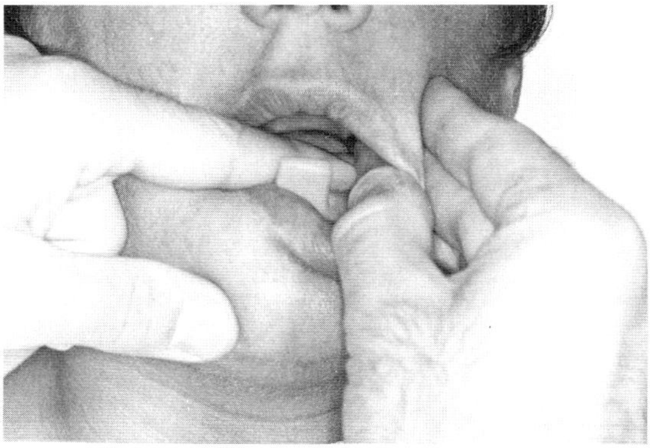

Fig. 5-10 The tray is held securely with one hand while the other hand draws the cheek up to bring excess compound onto the outer tray surface.

With the other hand, massage the lip from side to side (Fig. 5-12) to mold the compound to the desired functional extension. This moves the orbicularis oris muscle, along with its associated muscles of facial expression (Figs. 5-13a and b). The flange should extend to contact the mucous membrane reflection at rest and have sufficient thickness to restore the proper esthetic position of the lower lip. The patient can be instructed to pout (Fig. 5-14a) or to lick his lower lip with his tongue (Fig. 5-14b). Pouting activates the mentalis muscle; licking the lower lip activates the muscles of the lower lip as it moves.

Flame heat the area of the labial frenum. Temper and place it in the mouth. Register this area first by elevating the frenum into the compound and then by massaging the lip with a side-to-side motion. As was the case with the buccal frena, this action provides freedom of movement for the frenum itself while still maintaining functional contact with the adjacent tissues.

Retromylohyoid area

Flame heat the retromylohyoid area (Table 5-4) bilaterally and temper it. Place it in the mouth and hold the tray in position bilaterally. Instruct the patient to push his tongue against the tray handle. Reheat and retemper this area, and have the patient place his tongue into his right and left cheeks while the tray is held in position. With these actions, the

Table 5-2 Buccal flange and buccal frena areas

Anatomic region	Tissues that influence extension	How to activate	What activation accomplishes
Buccal flange	External oblique ridge Buccinator muscle	Manually manipulate the cheek with finger pressure upon the denture border in an anterior-posterior direction	Moves the fibers of the buccinator muscle and the soft tissues of the cheek in the direction of the muscle activity during patient function
		Look at the buccal flange internally to see that the cheek is not distended and the tissues of the cheek rest upon the outer surface of the dentures	Avoids overextension, which can cause displacement of the denture base and soreness of the tissues
		Feel the edge of the flange with the ball of the index finger to check for overextension	Avoids overextension, which can cause displacement of the denture base and soreness of the tissues
		Feel and observe the cheek from the outside of the mouth for overextension	Provides detection of overextension of border and visualization of esthetics and facial form
Buccal frena	Buccal frena	Elevate the frena into the compound and then mold the cheek in an anterior-posterior direction	Allows for freedom of movement of the connective tissue band Permits a seal to form by the manipulation of the cheek in a back-and-forth motion; therefore, allows maximum seal and contact with freedom of movement

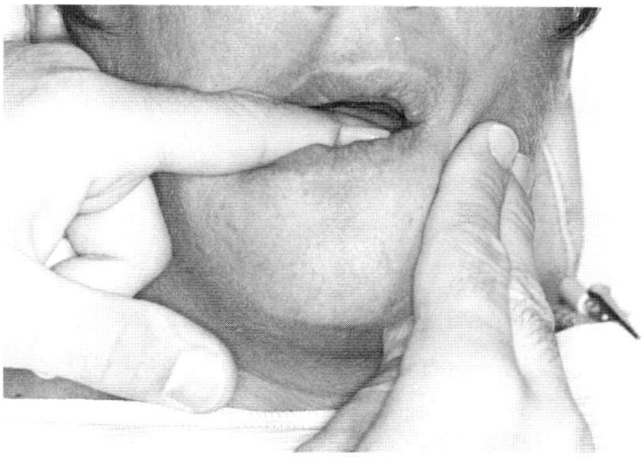

Fig. 5-11 The tray is held in position with one hand while the other molds the cheeks in an anterior-posterior direction using manual pressure against the compound.

Table 5-3 Labial flange and labial frenum areas

Anatomic region	Tisues that influence extension	How to activate	What activation accomplishes
Labial flange	Mentalis muscle Incisive labii inferioris Orbicularis oris with associated muscles of facial expression Labial frenum	Hand massage and manipulate the lip in a side-to-side motion	Activates the orbicularis oris muscle with its associated muscles of facial expression
		Instruct the patient to evert the lower lip (pout)	Activates the mentalis muscle against the compound
		Instruct the patient to lick the upper and lower lips with the tongue	Activates the orbicularis oris muscle and its associated muscles of facial expression
Labial frenum	Labial frenum and its associated connective tissue fibers	Elevate the frenum into the compound and then massage the lip with a side-to-side motion	Allows for freedom of movement of the connective tissue–formed frenum
			Permits a seal to form by the molding of the area using the side-to-side movement of the lip; therefore, maximum seal with freedom of movement

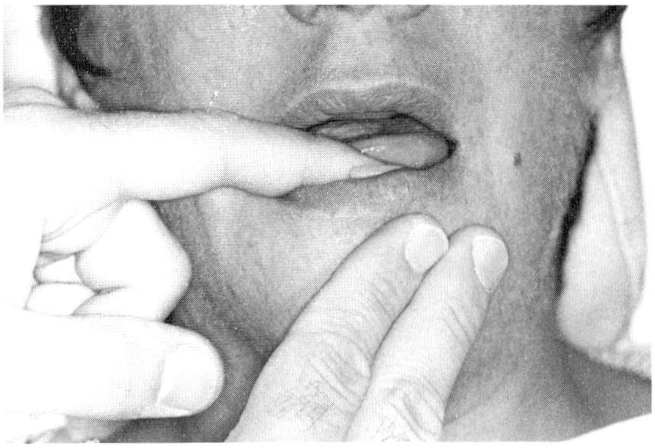

Fig. 5-12 The tray is held in position with one hand while the other moves the lip from side to side.

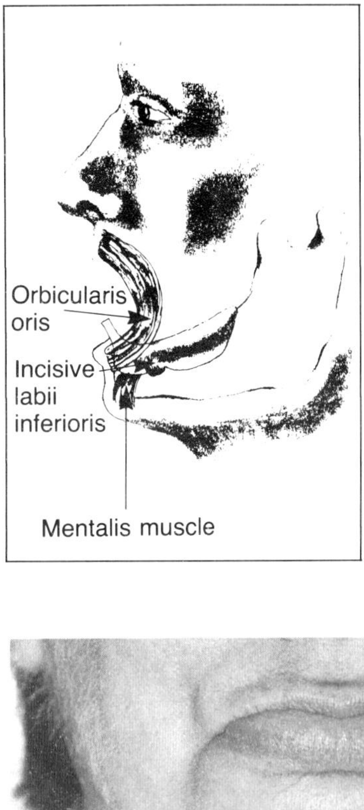

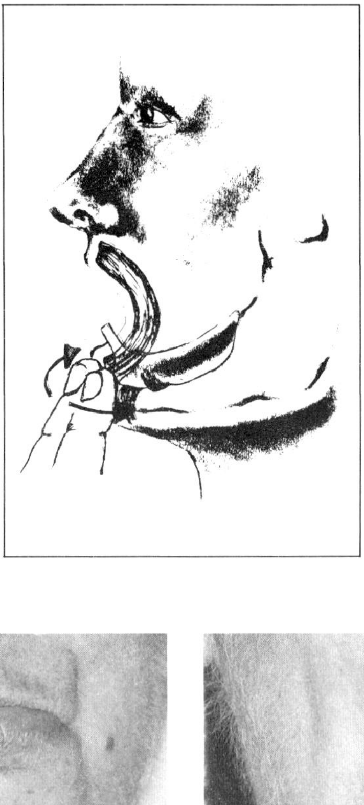

Figs. 5-13a *(left)* The muscles that limit the extension of the labial flange with the impression tray in position are shown.

Fig. 5-13b *(right)* The lip is manipulated side to side *(arrows)* to move these muscles.

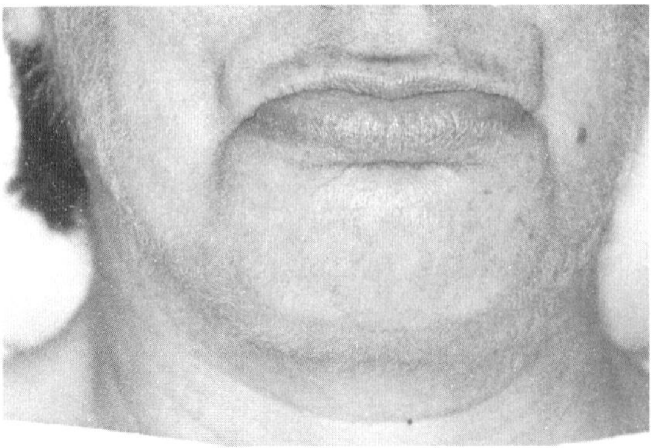

Fig. 5-14a The patient is instructed to pout (evert the lower lip)—this activates the mentalis muscle fibers.

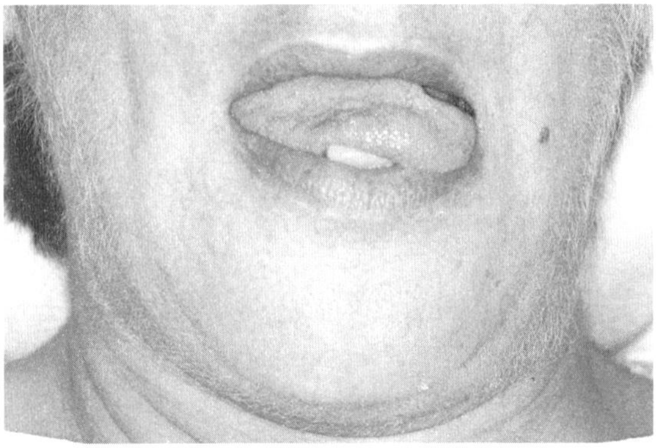

Fig. 5-14b The patient is instructed to lick his lower lip with his tongue—this activates the muscles of the lower lip.

Table 5-4 Retromolar area and retromylohyoid curtain

Anatomic region	Tissues that influence extension	How to activate	What activation accomplishes
Retromolar area and retromylohyoid curtain	Superior constrictor muscle Glossopalatine muscle	Instruct the patient to push his tongue against the handle and then bite down on your fingers on top of the handle	As the tongue is protruded against the handle with force, the superior constrictor muscle and the glossopalatine muscle contract and act against the denture border; as the patient bites down, the internal pterygoid muscle contracts and acts against the denture border
		Instruct the patient to move his tongue into his right and left cheeks while the tray is held in position	This tongue movement moves impression material so that the future tongue action will not displace the completed denture

superior constrictor and glossopalatine muscles contract and impress the overlying tissues against the impression compound (Fig. 5-15). These tongue movements displace excess compound from the borders so that the denture will not be unseated when the patient moves his tongue during function.

Mylohyoid area

Flame heat the mylohyoid area (Table 5-5) bilaterally. Temper and place the tray in the mouth. Hold the tray in position with both hands. Instruct the patient to place the tip of his tongue into the upper and lower vestibules on the right and left sides. Reheat the area again bilaterally and instruct the patient to swallow two or three times in rapid succession. The tongue movements raise the level of the floor of the mouth through contraction of the mylohyoid muscle (Figs. 5-16a and b). The amount of movement of the floor of the mouth may be greater with tongue movement than with swallowing. The swallowing action will sometimes allow the denture to extend further into the floor of the mouth for a peripheral seal. The repetitive swallowing usually allows the compound to extend further into the peripheral border areas than the tongue movements will permit. Individual variation is seen among patients. If significantly differ-

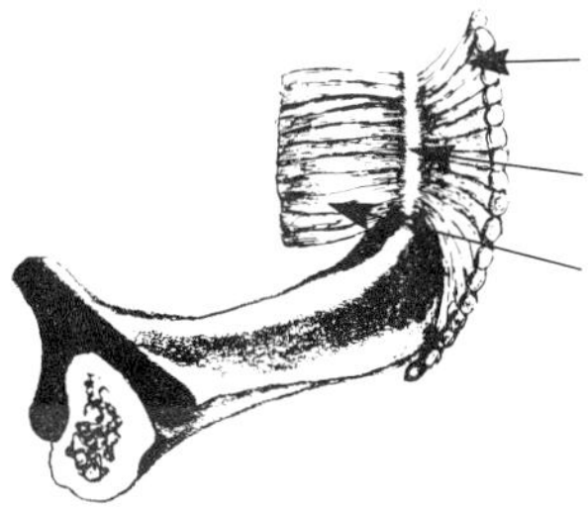

Fig. 5-15 The muscles that limit the extension of the retromylohyoid area are illustrated with the impression tray in place.

Table 5-5 Mylohyoid area

Anatomic region	Tissues that influence extension	How to activate	What activation accomplishes
Mylohyoid area	Mylohyoid muscle Mylohyoid ridge and the medial body of the mandible Tongue size, position, and amount of movement	Have the patient perform repetitive, forced swallowing	Causes a forcible contraction of the mylohyoid muscle fibers; moves the compound inferiorly and medially
		Instruct the patient to move his tongue into the upper and lower vestibules on each side of his mouth	Raises the floor of the mouth through contraction of the mylohyoid muscle. The amount of movement of the floor of the mouth is often greater with tongue movement. The swallowing activity, therefore, will sometimes allow the denture to extend further into the floor of the mouth for a better seal and better stabilization. If different configurations do exist, use the activity that provides the maximum extension compatible with function.
		Contour the border and the outer surface of the flange to pass under the tongue	The denture border can extend inferiorly and medially to the mylohyoid ridge so as to: • help prevent soreness of the tissues over the ridge • have the tongue rest upon the outer, polished surface of the denture to increase the stability of the denture

ent configurations result from the two different actions, select the function that provides for minimal extension so that the denture will not be dislodged during function.

The mylohyoid extension should be contoured laterally to pass under the tongue, inferiorly and medially to the mylohyoid ridge. The tongue will increase the stability of the denture as it rests upon the denture flange and border.

Sublingual fold space and lingual frenum

Place additional compound on the sublingual fold space and the lingual frenum area (Table 5-6). Flame heat, temper, and place the tray in the mouth. Seal this area to the greatest possible depth by placing your finger directly on the compound and pushing it in a downward and anterior direction until it is firm. Remove and chill in ice water.

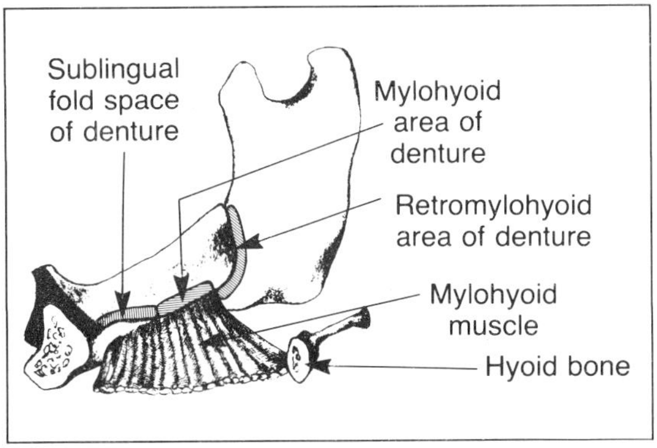

Fig. 5-16a The muscles that limit the extension of the mylohyoid area are illustrated with the impression tray in place.

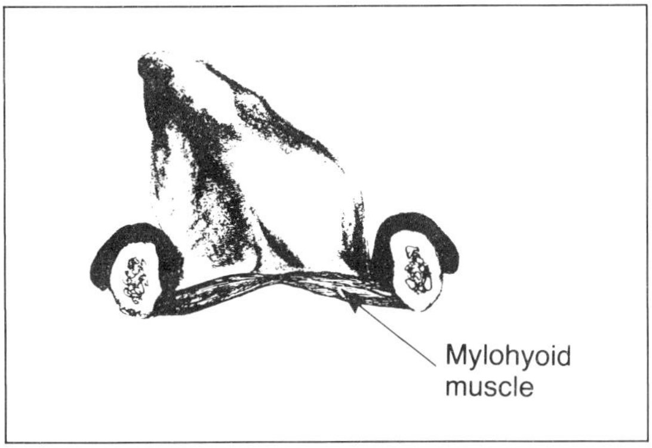

Fig. 5-16b Elevating the tongue raises the level of the floor of the mouth and causes contraction of the mylohyoid muscle.

Reheat the surface of this area, temper, and reinsert the tray. This area is functionally molded by having the patient move his tongue forward to the tray handle and wet his upper and lower lips with the tip of his tongue. These functional movements cause slight contraction of the genioglossus muscle, which pushes against the tissues superior to it (see Fig. 1-14).

Only slight function of the genioglossus muscle is required, so that the lingual flange in this area can be gradually reduced until the most favorable level—that which provides for peripheral seal and tongue function—is reached. The mylohyoid muscle is activated when the tongue is elevated, but its effect is more limited in this area because it is inferior to the geniohyoid muscle and the soft tissues above it. The lingual flange in this area is reduced and contoured by these functional movements until the most favorable level is reached. The goal is to provide for a maximum of soft tissue placement for a peripheral seal yet still allow freedom of tongue movement and patient comfort. Do not overshorten; if you do, the seal and therefore the retention may be lost. If a prominent or active lingual frenum is present, heat the lingual frenum area and have the patient protrude his tongue and then move it side to side to register that narrowly defined area *only*.

Check the retention of the impression by having the patient move his tongue and mandible within the range of average function. At this point the impression should have good retention and stability if the prognosis was favorable for each (as discussed in chapter 1). Also, lift the tray handle anteriorly. If the impression is not retentive, check the sublingual fold space and the masseteric notch areas. Lengthen the sublingual fold space area first, as described earlier. If not sufficient, try modifying the extension into the masseteric notch area to fit the undersurface of the buccal fat pad to a closer extent. The border seal in the sublingual fold space is crucial to the overall retention of the mandibular complete denture base. If this area is not sealed, a significant decrease in retention can result. As mentioned in chapter 2, tongue position plays an important role in the anatomic form that the sublingual fold space will assume. Also check the masseteric notch area to see that a seal has formed and that the buccal fat pad is positioned correctly. Once these procedures are accomplished, the impression is complete (Fig. 5-17).

Finally, box the impression in such a way as to preserve the width of the periphery as well as the length of the flange. Pour a stone cast.

Problems

Many philosophies and techniques for impression making have been advocated. Yet we continue to see an overwhelming number of mandibular dentures that do not adequately or properly cover the

Table 5-6 Sublingual fold space and lingual frenum areas

Anatomic region	Tissues that influence extension	How to activate	What activation accomplishes
Sublingual fold space (last area to be border molded)	Genioglossus muscle Tongue (with its associated intrinsic and extrinsic musculature) Lingual frenum Folds of mucosa covering the genioglossus muscle and sublingual glands Mylohyoid muscle	Place additional compound into this area. Seal this area to its lowest level by massaging the compound downward with the index finger. Surface heat and gradually shorten this area by having the tongue just contact the handle of the tray to prevent reduction of the length too rapidly.	Causes slight contraction of the genioglossus muscle, which pushes against the tissues superior to it. Only mild activation of the genioglossus muscle is accomplished, so that the lingual flange in this area is gradually reduced until the most favorable level—that which provides for peripheral seal and tongue function—is reached. The mylohyoid muscle is activated when the tongue is elevated, but its effect is more limited in this area because it is inferior to the geniohyoid muscle and the soft tissues above it.
		Instruct the patient to gently wet his upper and lower lips with his tongue	Same as above
Lingual frenum	Lingual frenum with its intrinsic connective tissue fibers	Instruct the patient to protrude his tongue slightly and move it from side to side. Make sure that the compound is warmed only in the area to be contacted by the lingual frenum.	Allows freedom of the lingual frenum connective tissue band to prevent the denture from being dislodged during normal tongue movements

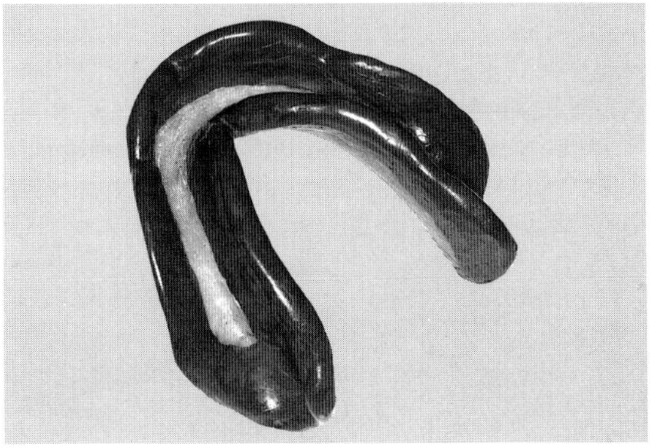

Fig. 5-17 The completed mandibular impression.

appropriate tissues. Inadequate impressions are often made of the following areas. As a result, the completed bases do not adequately cover the tissues of *(1)* the retromolar pad, *(2)* the buccal shelf–supporting area, *(3)* the masseteric notch area, and *(4)* the sublingual fold space.

Summary

A custom tray with peripheral relief is used to make a selective tissue placement impression. The impression tray is rigid, properly contoured for each patient, and practical to use. The tray can be positioned in the mouth the same way with each insertion. The unrelieved resin surfaces cover a large tissue area to act as a positive stop and seat for the custom tray. The custom tray gives excellent support in height and width to the compound during border molding.

The custom tray with peripheral relief offers a method to control the amount of tissue placement that is applied to the various denture-bearing tissues. The principle of selective tissue placement is applied here, because the alginate impression material is used to record the attached mucosa with minimal placement, while compound is used to record the movable tissues and peripheral sulcus with additional placement. The slopes of the ridges are primary supporting and bearing areas, and they are functionally loaded with the compound during the molding of the final impression.

Through the use of compound, areas may be built up or reduced to develop maximum retention and stability in the final impression. The stability and retention of the impression can be tested prior to final completion.

The degree of retention and stability of a mandibular denture can be predicted. Very positive retention and stability can still be provided for many patients who have "no ridge" and a flat floor of the mouth.

Allen Brewer
(Personal communication)

Chapter 6

Maxillary Final Impression

The maxillary final impression described in this chapter is accomplished using the same type of custom tray used for the mandibular impression (chapter 5). The impression tray has an unrelieved area on the crest of the ridge and a relieved area on the slopes of the ridges and the peripheral border (Fig. 6-1, see also Fig. 4-1). As with the mandibular impression, the unrelieved area of the tray is intimately adapted to the crest of the ridge. Because no impression material is ever added to this area, it provides a stable and controlled position to which the impression tray is repeatedly returned while the final impression is being made. Therefore, the borders can be changed as necessary (compound can be added and removed) until the desired impression is obtained. The relieved area, on the other hand, is the space in which the impression compound is added. The making of the impression in this manner enables the dentist to produce a selective tissue placement impression without the use of a wash impression material such as zinc oxide–eugenol or rubber base within the border-molded tray.

Border molding is described in this chapter by detailing *(1)* the hard and soft tissues that mold the compound in each peripheral border area, *(2)* the techniques that the dentist and patient can use to activate the tissues for each border area, and *(3)* the muscular or tissue movements that each of these techniques accomplishes.

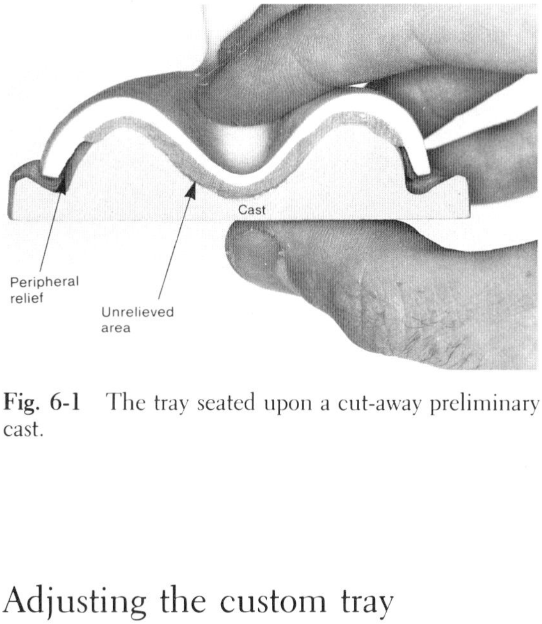

Fig. 6-1 The tray seated upon a cut-away preliminary cast.

Adjusting the custom tray

The custom tray is adjusted and the impression is made using the guidelines already presented for the six areas that were defined to anatomically trim the preliminary alginate impression (Fig. 6-2).

The objectives of adjusting the impression tray at this time are *(1)* to trim the peripheral borders so that they are 2 to 3 mm short of the ultimate denture borders, and *(2)* to achieve a tray that has the appearance of the completed impression.

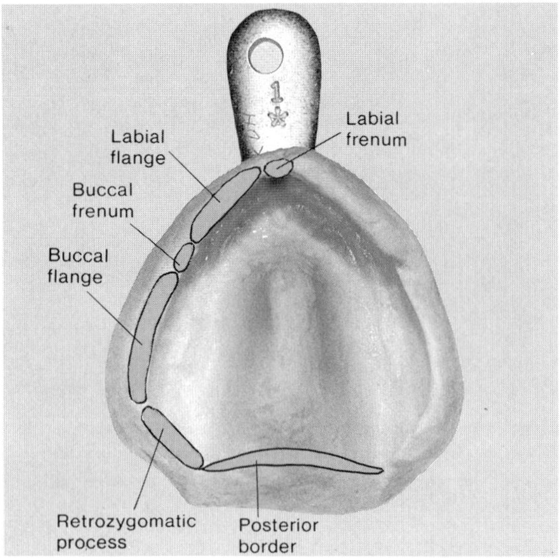

Fig. 6-2 The maxillary denture base has been divided into six anatomic areas. The preliminary alginate impression was trimmed using these areas for reference; likewise, the final impression is completed using the same guidelines.

Trimming the impression tray

Place the impression tray in the patient's mouth and examine it. Then adjust it where indicated, area by area, as follows.

Retrozygomatic area

This is usually the extension with the greatest width. The tray should not be thinned excessively here because it would then be difficult to capture the proper width of the border. The compound must not only be supported in height but also in width. This factor is often overlooked in the fabrication of impression trays. Many maxillary impression trays are made with knife-edged borders that do not adequately support the border-molding material used. Place the ball of your index finger in the retrozygomatic area and instruct the patient to close. Closing will cause the coronoid process to move posteriorly and allow you to feel the extension of the impression tray. The tray should be slightly (1 to 2 mm) short of the intended extension.

Coronoid process area

Trim this area so as to allow room for the coronoid process as the mandible moves from side to side and opens wide. Thin the tray in this area from the height of the flange to the outer surface of the custom tray opposite the tuberosity.

Zygomatic area

Trim this area to be thinner than the retrozygomatic area. The width of the tray becomes progressively thinner proceeding anteriorly up to the buccal frena. Palpation with the ball of your index finger is helpful in determining the appropriate extension. The impression tray should be approximately 2 to 3 mm short of the periphery. The cheek can also be reflected so the border position of the tray can be visualized. The tray is relieved to allow freedom of movement for the buccal frena.

Labial flange and labial frenum areas

Trim these areas to be thinner than the retrozygomatic and zygomatic areas, though not knife edged. The border should be rounded, with an average thickness of approximately 2 mm. Reflect the lip to visualize the tray length as it relates to the height of the peripheral sulcus (Fig. 6-3). Also palpate the outer surface of the lip and cheeks to ensure that there is no overextension. The lip and cheeks should feel flat. Bulky border extensions affect esthetics. Step back and look at the patient's lips to make certain that the tray does not adversely protrude the facial tissues.

Adjust the labial frena until there is no interference when the frenum is manually manipulated in any functional direction (Fig. 6-4).

Posterior palatal seal area

Trim the posterior extent of the tray to just reach the "vibrating line," the imaginary line indicating the beginning of motion of the soft palate. The vibrating line should be delineated by having the patient say "ah" and locating the approximate junction of movement. Use an intraoral marking pencil to mark the junction (Fig. 6-5).

Continue the line through the hamular notches on each side. The tray can be inserted into the mouth and checked accordingly.

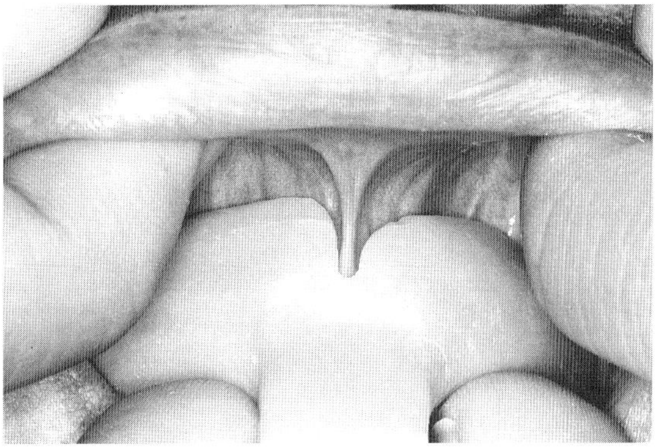

Fig. 6-3 Reflect the lips to see that there is adequate room on the labial flange area to add compound.

Making the maxillary final impression

Impression compound is now methodically added to the relieved areas and to the periphery. It is perfected in two stages: *(1)* the initial adaptation of the compound, and *(2)* the border molding to completion of the final impression.

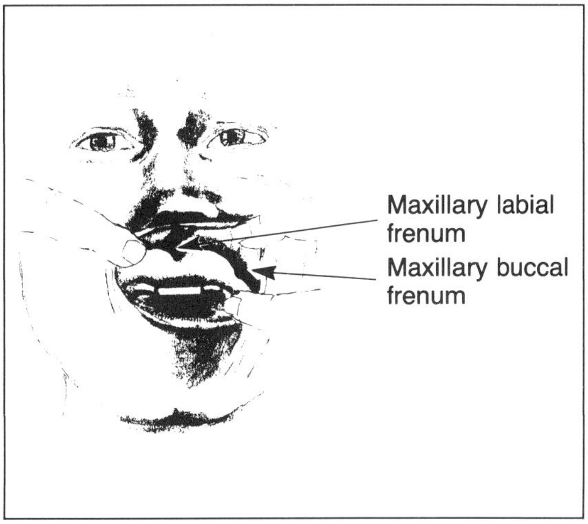

Fig. 6-4 Adjust the labial frena until there is no interference when the lip is manipulated normally.

Initial adaptation of the compound

1. Use the flame from a Bunsen burner to soften the end of a stick of impression compound. Generously fill all the relieved areas of the tray up to the butt joint with compound (Fig. 6-6). Place additional compound around the entire periphery.
2. Use the flame from an alcohol torch to soften the compound on the tray, and dip the tray in a water bath at the working temperature of the compound to temper and evenly soften the compound.
3. Place the tray in the patient's mouth and seat it slowly, allowing the compound to flow (Fig. 6-7). Repeat steps 1, 2, and 3 until the compound has flowed over the entire butt joint and filled all areas of the relieved portion of the tray. If voids exist, add more compound. This may involve several trial insertions.
4. Remove the tray from the patient's mouth and chill it in ice water. Scrape the excess compound back to the butt joint using a small vulcanite scraper, being careful not to mar the acrylic resin tray. Also remove any excess material that has flowed onto the outer surface of the tray.
5. Reheat the compound and repeat steps 3 and 4 until no compound covers the unrelieved portion of the tray. This unrelieved area of the tray already represents the final impression of the tissue which it covers. No wash impression will be made over it. Therefore, only the relieved areas need to be impressioned and border molded.

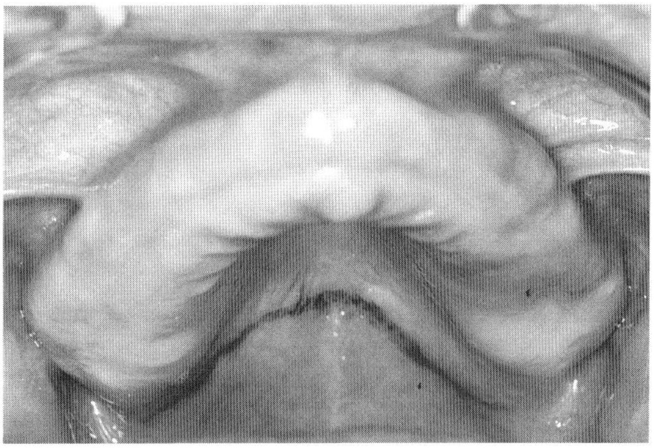

Fig. 6-5 Mark the vibrating line on the palate.

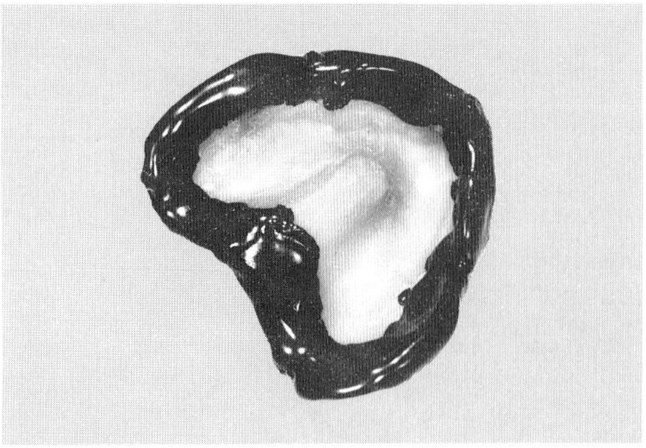

Fig. 6-6 All the relieved areas of the custom tray are filled generously with compound.

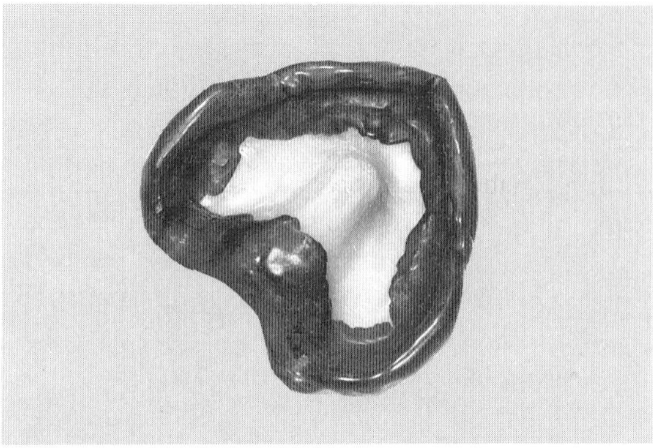

Fig. 6-7 Excess compound has flowed over the butt joint onto the unrelieved portion of the tray.

Border molding and completing the impression

Retrozygomatic and coronoid process areas

Dry the compound and flame heat the retrozygomatic areas (Table 6-1) on both sides. Temper and place the impression in the mouth while it is partially closed to allow the compound to occupy this potential space without being blocked by the coronoid process. Instruct the patient to pull in with his lips on your finger. The patient's cheek can also be manually manipulated in an anterior-posterior direction (Fig. 6-8). Use the ball of your index finger to push warmed compound up into the retrozygomatic area before functioning the patient. This area of the denture base is easily underextended. It is important to adequately extend impression material in this area for retention. Remove the tray and chill it in ice water. Flame heat the coronoid process area on both sides and insert. Instruct the patient to close and to move his mandible from side to side, then immediately ask the patient to open wide (Fig. 6-9). The side-to-side motion records the activity of the coronoid process in a closed position, whereas opening causes the coronoid process to sweep past the denture periphery (Figs. 6-10a to d). It is sometimes necessary to reheat and reactivate this area several times to record the effect of the coronoid process.

Zygomatic areas and buccal frena

Flame heat the compound in the zygomatic area, (Table 6-2) bilaterally. Temper and insert it into the mouth. Manually mold the cheek in an anterior-posterior direction using slight finger pressure against the compound, or tell the patient to suck on your finger. Remove the compound and chill in ice water. Flame heat the buccal frenum area on one side. Temper and insert it into the patient's mouth. Manually mold the cheeks and the frenum, first downward into the compound, then in an anterior-posterior direction. Remove and chill, then heat the opposite side for the same activity.

Labial flange and labial frenum area

Flame heat the labial flange area (Table 6-3) bilaterally. Temper and insert it in the mouth. Manually mold the compound by externally moving the lip in a side-to-side direction while simultaneously applying finger pressure to control the width of the border (Figs. 6-11a and b). Remove and chill in the water. Flame heat the labial frenum. Temper and insert it in the mouth. Lift the patient's upper lip and vertically place the frenum into the softened compound; then immediately mold with your fingers using a side-to-side external motion. Again use slight manual pressure to mold the compound. Esthetics play a dominant role in the width of this border. Compound can be added or removed as necessary to achieve the desired facial support.

Table 6-1 Retrozygomatic and coronoid process areas

Anatomic region	Tissues that mold	How to activate	What activation accomplishes
Retrozygomatic area	Buccinator muscle fibers and overlying mucosa	Manually push softened compound into the retrozygomatic area with the ball of your index finger; the patient's mouth should be closed	Enables compound to occupy this space, which is often blocked by the coronoid process
		Instruct the patient to pull in on your finger with his lips, and manipulate the cheek in an anterior-posterior and downward direction	Activates the buccinator muscle fibers and moves the overlying mucosa
		Instruct the patient to close firmly against your fingers	Causes the masseter muscles to contract against the modeling plastic
Coronoid process area	Coronoid process Fibers of the temporal muscle attached to the coronoid process	Instruct the patient to open wide then close and move his mandible to the opposite side	Activates the coronoid process and the attached fibers of the temporal muscle against the modeling plastic

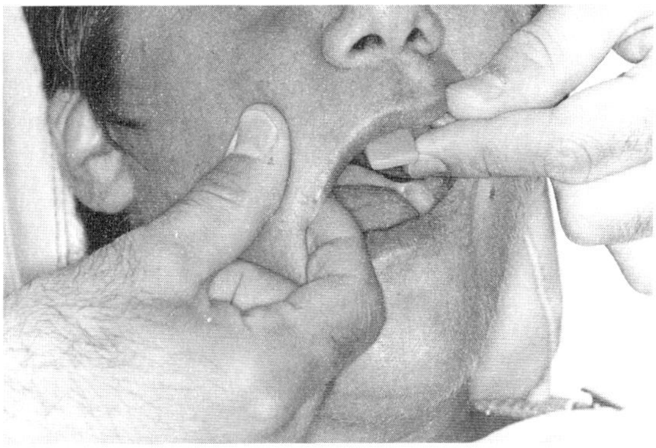

Fig. 6-8 Manually manipulate the patient's cheek in an anterior-posterior direction.

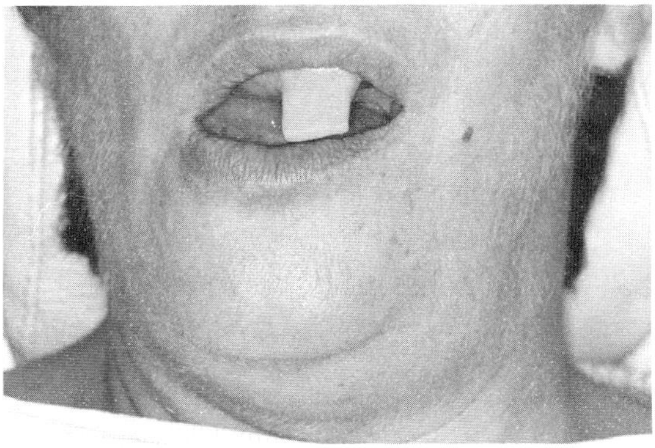

Fig. 6-9 Instruct the patient to move his mandible from side to side while his mouth is slightly open. Then immediately have the patient open his mouth fully.

Figs. 6-10a to d As the mandible moves side to side while the mouth is in a relatively closed position, and then as the mouth is opened wide, the coronoid process will mold the compound.

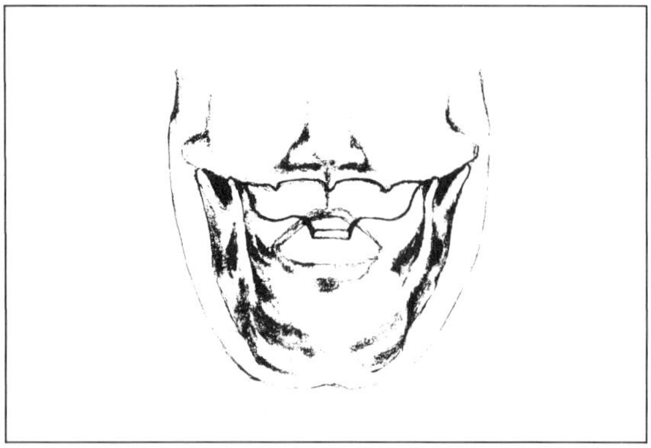

Fig. 6-10a

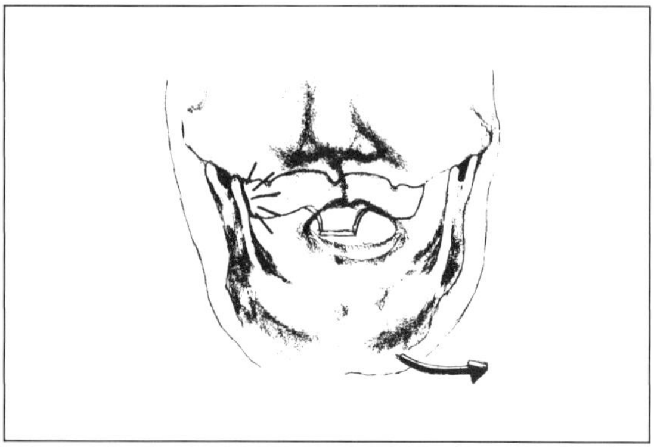

Fig. 6-10b

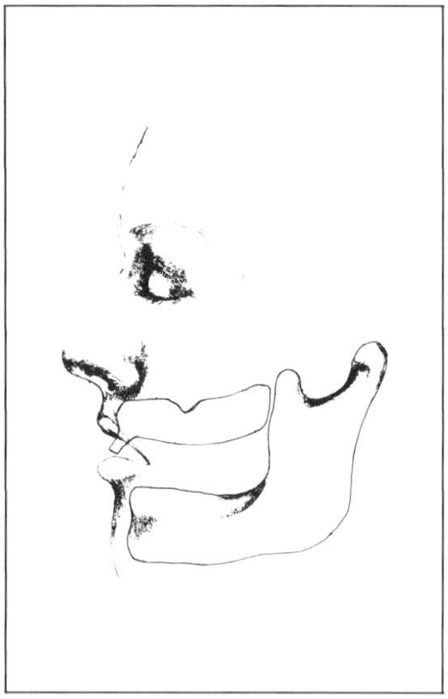

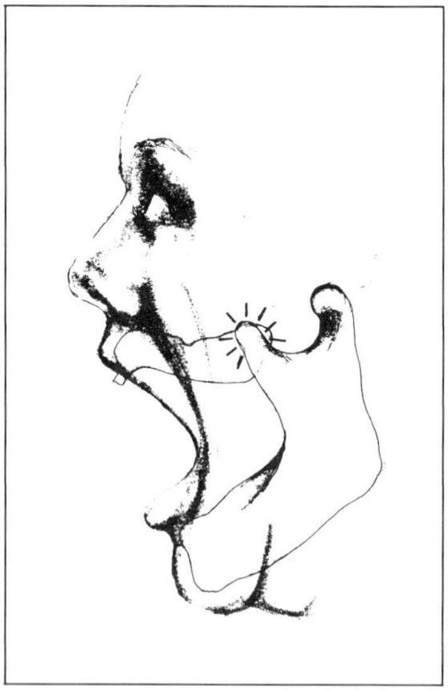

Fig. 6-10c *(left)*

Fig. 6-10d *(right)*

Table 6-2 Zygomatic and buccal frena areas

Anatomic region	Tissues that mold	How to activate	What activation accomplishes
Zygomatic area or buccal flange	Buccinator muscle Zygomaticomaxillary crest Buccal frena and associated muscles of facial expression	Manually mold the cheek in a side-to-side direction. Instruct the patient to pull his cheeks in on your finger. Also instruct the patient to move his jaw from side to side to have the coronoid process mold the compound.	Simulates the movement of the buccinator muscle and associated soft tissues; the lip movement causes the buccinator muscle to contract. Improves esthetic form of lips and cheeks.
		Add or remove compound to allow the impression to fulfill esthetic requirements. Muscles do not exert a dominant role in the width of this denture border.	Aids in determining and limiting the flange length. Also, improves esthetic form of lips and cheeks.
Buccal frena	Buccal frena with associated connective tissue fibers and the muscles of facial expression, particularly the caninus muscle and the orbicularis oris muscle, which affect the frena movement	Pull the buccal frena	Activates the connective tissue fibers of the frena while simultaneously causing movement of the associated muscles of facial expression (caninus and orbicularis oris muscles)

Table 6-3 Labial flange and labial frenum areas

Anatomic region	Tissues that mold	How to activate	What activation accomplishes
Labial flange	Orbicularis oris Quadratus labii inferioris (superior incisive muscles) Risorius	Mold this area externally using your fingers to move the lip back and forth while simultaneously applying pressure to control the width of the border	Manually manipulates the lips with their associated musculature to seal the denture border in displaceable tissue; the pressure helps control the esthetic form of the peripheral roll
		Instruct the patient to lick his upper lip; do this with only the surface of the compound heated	Moves the orbicularis oris in a common activity
		Observe esthetics	Causes compound to be added or removed to conform to esthetic considerations
Labial frenum	Labial frenum	Lift the upper lip vertically, place the frenum into the compound, and then manually mold this area externally by moving the lip while simultaneously applying pressure to control the width of the area	Manually manipulates the tissue of the frenum in the compound to give it freedom to function; the pressure ensures both a seal in the displaceable tissue and esthetic form

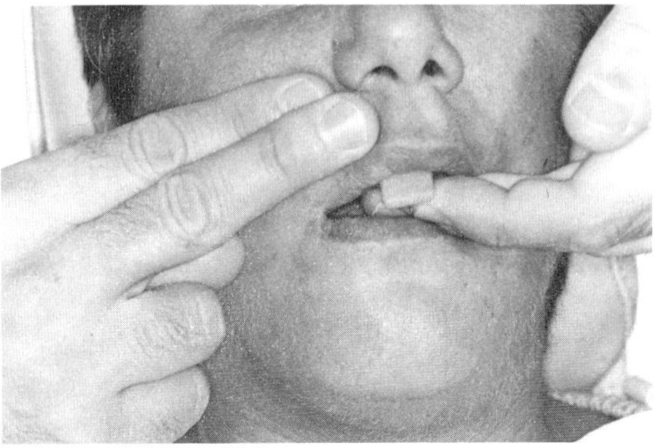

Fig. 6-11a Mold the lip in a side-to-side direction using slight finger pressure.

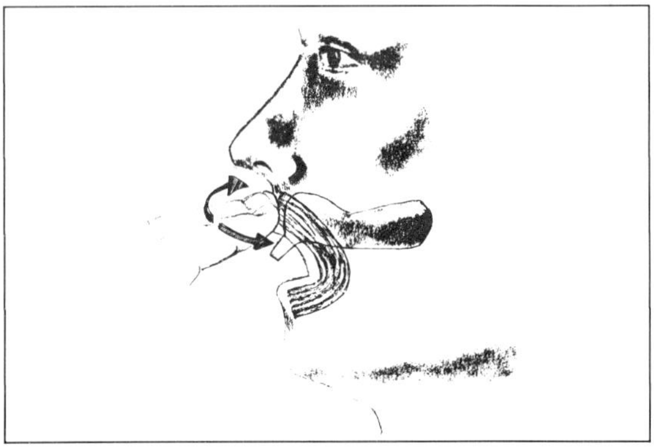

Fig. 6-11b This activity manipulates the lip and the underlying orbicularis oris muscle.

Table 6-4 Posterior palatal seal area

Anatomic region	Tissues that mold	How to activate	What activation accomplishes
Posterior palatal seal area	Pterygomaxillary raphe Pterygoid hamulus and hamular notch Palatopharyngeus muscle Palatoglossus muscle Tensor veli palatini muscle Levator veli palatini muscle	Instruct the patient to open wide Hold the patient's nostrils closed with your fingers; instruct the patient to blow through his nose Add an additional layer of compound and insert and have the patient swallow	Causes the pterygomaxillary raphe to become more taut Causes the soft palate to depress against the modeling plastic through the contraction of the tensor veli palatini, delineating the junction of the hard and soft palate Displaces the posterior palatal tissues superiorly with only minimal downward pressure by the tensor veli palatini

Posterior palatal seal area

Flame heat the posterior palatal seal area (Table 6-4) from hamular notch to hamular notch. Temper and insert it in the mouth. Instruct the patient to open wide and to protrude his mandible to make an impression of the pterygomaxillary raphe and anterior border of the ramus, respectively. Remove, chill, and dry the compound. The "vibrating line" should again be located by having the patient say "ah." Use a disposable marker* to mark the junction of movement. Then insert the denture in the patient's mouth to determine the location of the posterior extension. If the impression extends too far posteriorly, the ink mark will be covered and transferred to the impression. If the impression is too short posteriorly, the ink mark will be visible.

*Dr. Thompson's Color Transfer Applicators, Great Plains Dental Products Co., Kingman, Kan.

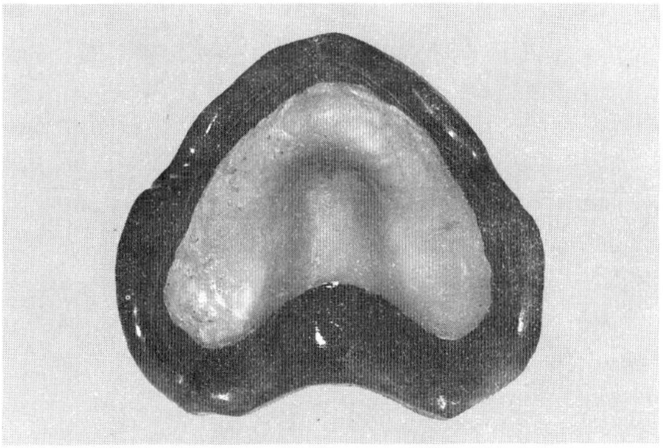

Fig. 6-12 The completed impression.

Add or remove compound where indicated to finalize the most posterior extension.

If a favorable prognosis was made initially (see chapter 1), the impression should now have good retention and stability. Additional retention may sometimes be achieved by adding a second layer of compound or fluid wax to the posterior palatal seal area (Fig. 6-12).

Box the impression, preserving the width of the periphery as well as the length of the flanges. Pour a stone cast.

Common impressioning errors in maxillary dentures

The most common errors that occur in making maxillary dentures are described as follows.

Border extensions for support and retention

The borders do not extend to the functionally available area for support and retention—they are either over- or underextended in height and/or width. The purpose of a functionally border-molded and properly extended denture base is to create a denture that is physiologically and esthetically adapted to the tissues in function and at rest. When a person speaks, chews, swallows, yawns, whistles, wets his lips, or opens and closes his mouth, the peripheral border tissues move. The tissues are constantly changing their shape, location, and tension. Thus, if an impression is not functionally adapted or adequately extended, the denture will likely lack stability and/or retention.

Border extensions and the coronoid process

The functional movements of the coronoid process can cause the denture to be dislodged or cause soreness if the borders are overextended.

Border extensions and esthetics

Overextended or underextended areas can cause the maxilla to appear unesthetic because of too much or too little bulk of the denture base material in the labial region. Too much bulk can also be uncomfortable for a patient.

Border extensions and comfort

A properly extended denture base extends the denture over a large area to increase the surface area of support and thus both stability and retention. Appropriately extended denture borders have varying thicknesses. Many dentures have thin, knife-edged borders throughout. An arbitrarily determined denture border could be discernible to the tongue or peripheral tissue areas and therefore be a source of patient discomfort. A functionally molded and properly extended border makes the peripheries of a denture blend well with the oral tissues. The proper extension and contour of the posterior palatal seal area of the maxillary denture base are important for this region. Otherwise, food and saliva can easily get under the denture, causing discomfort and possible dislodgement of the denture.

Border extensions and frena

The area of frena attachments is often either under- or overextended. Overextended frena areas are a common cause of soreness. Overrelief of a frenum area can decrease retention.

Summary

A custom tray with peripheral relief is used to make a selective tissue placement impression. The impression tray is rigid, properly contoured for each patient, and efficient to use. The tray can be placed in the mouth in the same position with each insertion. The unrelieved resin surfaces cover a large tissue surface to act as a positive stop and seat for the custom tray. The custom tray gives excellent support in height and width to the compound during border molding.

The tray offers a means of controlling the amount of tissue placement of the various denture-bearing tissues. The principle of selective placement is applied here, because the alginate impression material is used to record the attached mucosa with minimal placement, while compound is used to record the movable tissues and peripheral sulcus with additional placement. The slopes of the ridges are primary supporting and bearing areas, and they are functionally loaded with the compound during the molding of the final impression.

Through the use of compound, areas may be built up or reduced to develop maximum retention and stability in the final impression. The stability and retention of the impression can be tested after completion.

The complexity of a procedure does not necessarily enhance the value of the result. Also, the person who is really wrong is the one who says, "Follow me, this is the only way to do it."

Allen Brewer
(Personal communication)

Chapter 7

Completed Denture Bases and Mounting Casts

Completed denture bases involve making heat-cured record bases immediately after the final impressions are made.[1,2] Jaw relation records and the try-in of the trial teeth are accomplished on these bases, which are the actual foundation of the future finished denture. A completed base, usually made of heat-cured acrylic resin, is the denture base that the patient will ultimately wear. This process requires that the denture teeth be processed to this existing base during a subsequent flasking procedure (Fig. 7-1).

In contrast to a completed base, a temporary base is defined as a trial record base that is used to make jaw relation records and to set teeth for the try-in appointment. A temporary denture base is most often made from shellac or autopolymerizing acrylic resin. It is discarded during the later flasking and processing steps for the final denture base.

This chapter will detail the techniques and rationale for using completed acrylic resin bases. Because the final impression cast is destroyed when the completed acrylic resin base is deflasked, the method for making mounting casts will be described. All of the materials needed for making completed denture bases and mounting casts are already available to the laboratory technician.

Technique for waxing a completed maxillary base

1. Flow a thin layer of melted baseplate wax onto the entire surface of the cast (Fig. 7-2). This wax will help the other wax to adhere to the cast. Add extra baseplate wax in the deep middle portions of the palate and in the valleys between the rugae. These areas of the denture base may be too thin because the sheet of baseplate wax to be added may be stretched and thinned as it is adapted to the cast.

2. Place strips of soft utility wax in the roll of the peripheral borders to maintain the appropriate thicknesses of the denture borders as captured in the final impression. Add the wax up to the crest of the ridges (Fig. 7-3). Do not place utility wax on the posterior palatal seal area.

3. Warm one sheet of baseplate wax (approximately 1 mm thick) over a flame, then manually adapt it over the entire cast and over the utility wax up to the land area (Fig. 7-4).

4. Cut the excess wax that passes onto the land area using a sharp blade. Seal the wax to the land area with a hot spatula.

5. Place a second layer of warmed baseplate wax in the palatal region of the maxillary cast (Fig. 7-5). This added wax serves two purposes: *(1)* it provides an external finishing line for the wax-up of the denture teeth to the processed base, and *(2)* it provides added rigidity to the completed base. The anterior portion of the finishing line is kept posterior to the rugae area. This will allow room to later customize the rugae onto the denture base during the final wax-up.

6. Add additional baseplate wax to extend the wax-up of the denture base over the back edge of the cast (Fig. 7-6). This wax is added to help minimize the anterior and superior shrinkage of the acrylic resin, as suggested by Vig.[3]

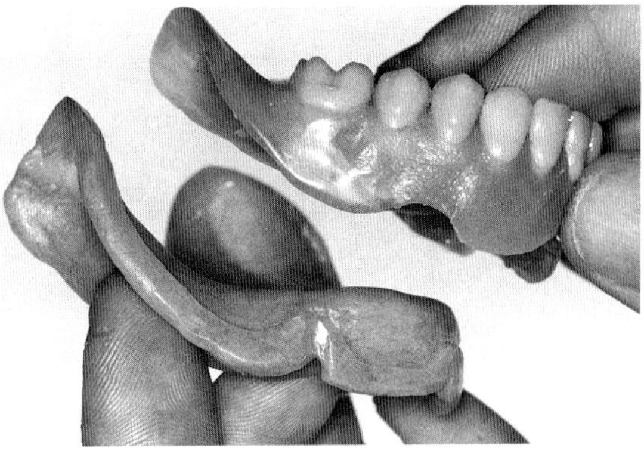

Fig. 7-1 The denture teeth with gingiva *(top)* and a completed denture base *(bottom)* to be added to the completed base during subsequent processing.

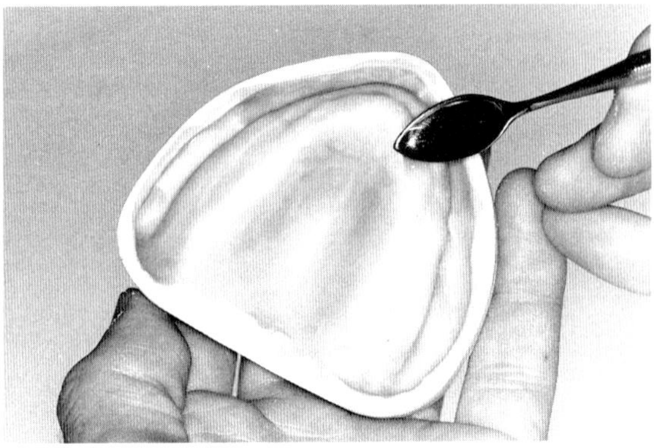

Fig. 7-2 A thin layer of melted baseplate wax is flowed onto the entire surface of the cast. It is particularly important to flow additional wax into the deep portions of the palate and into the valleys of the rugae.

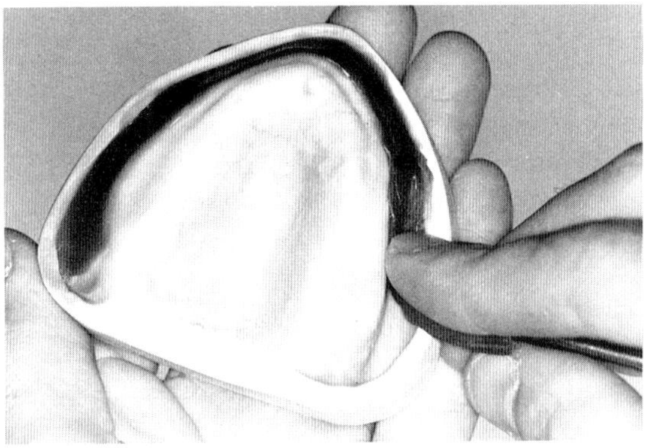

Fig. 7-3 Utility wax ropes are used to fill the denture border areas up to the crest of the ridge.

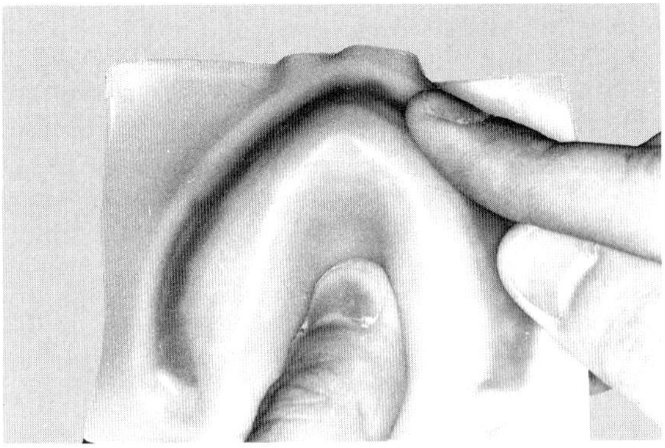

Fig. 7-4 One sheet of baseplate wax (approximately 1 mm thick) is adapted to the entire cast up to the land area.

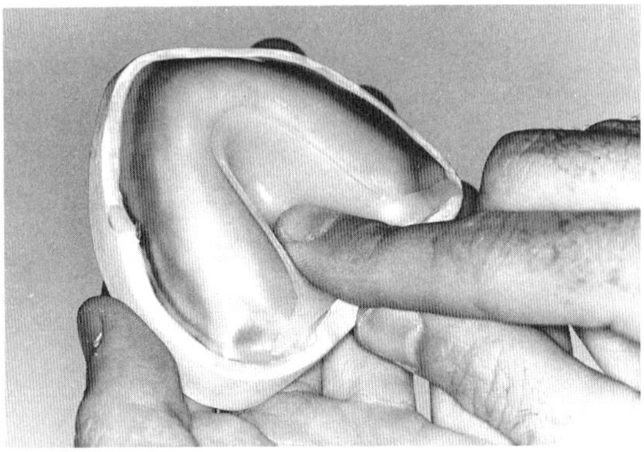

Fig. 7-5 A second layer of baseplate wax is cut out and added onto the posterior portion of the palate.

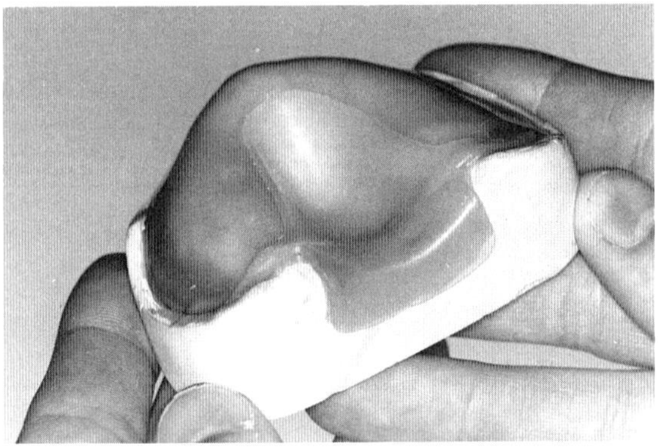

Fig. 7-6 The wax-up of the denture base is extended over the back edge of the cast.

Technique for waxing a completed mandibular base

The wax-up for the completed mandibular base is the same as for the completed maxillary base with two exceptions: *(1)* no additional sheet of baseplate wax is added over the initial baseplate wax, and *(2)* no wax is added over the posterior heels of the cast. The waxing technique for the completed mandibular base is illustrated in Figs. 7-7 to 7-9.

All undercuts in the outer surface of the wax-up should be filled with additional wax. If there is an undercut, it will make it more difficult to deflask the denture after processing. If excessive ridge resorption has occurred, additional wax should be added to the lingual aspect of the cast to ensure that the base will be rigid.

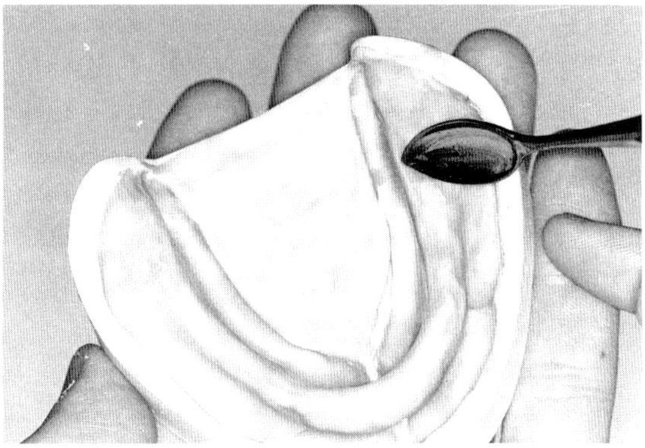

Fig. 7-7 A thin layer of melted baseplate wax is flowed onto the entire surface of the cast.

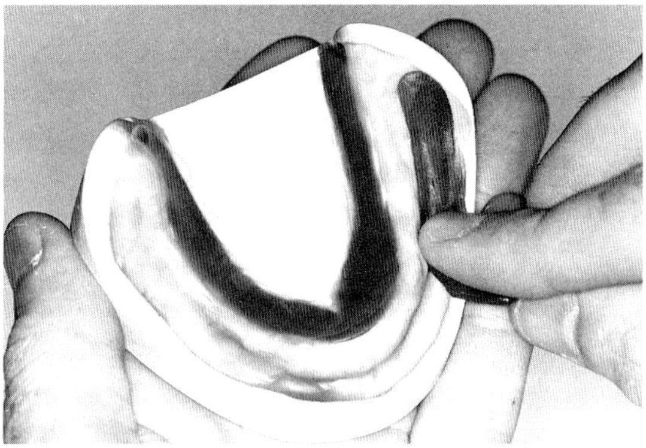

Fig. 7-8 Utility wax ropes are used to fill the denture border areas up to the crest of the ridge.

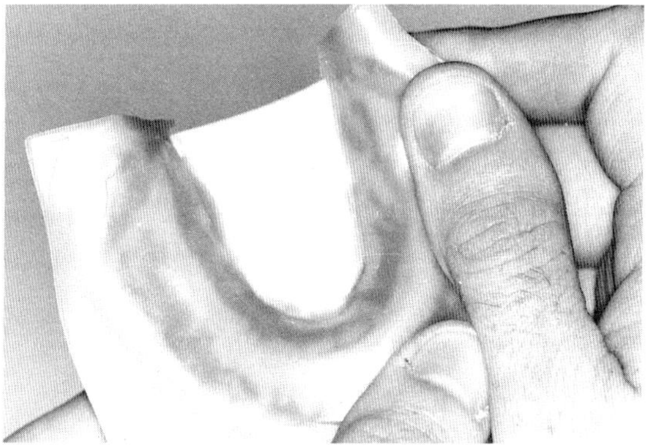

Fig. 7-9 One sheet of baseplate wax (approximately 1 mm thick) is adapted to the entire cast up to the land area.

Flasking and packing the waxed-up maxillary and mandibular bases

1. Lubricate the stone surfaces of the cast with a thin layer of petroleum jelly. This will allow for easy separation of the cast during deflasking.
2. Mix stone or plaster and invest the cast into the lower member of the flask (Figs. 7-10a and b). (Stone and slurry water can be used to accelerate the set of the stone.) Place the stone up to the land area of the cast, and remove and smooth the excess stone so that no undercuts exist. Flow melted baseplate wax onto the undercut or steep areas of stone so that the two halves of the flask will separate easily after the boilout. Place a thin layer of petroleum jelly on all stone surfaces as a separating medium.
3. Place the upper portion of the flask onto the lower member and vibrate another mix of stone into the flask. Put the top cap of the flask into place so stone releases from the top escape holes. Allow the stone to set for 30 minutes. A mixture of stone and slurry, if utilized, will set much faster (in approximately ten minutes) depending upon the concentration of slurry.
4. Place the flask in a large metal pan and pour boiling water into the pan until the water completely covers the surfaces of the flask. Remove the flask in five minutes and open it using a laboratory

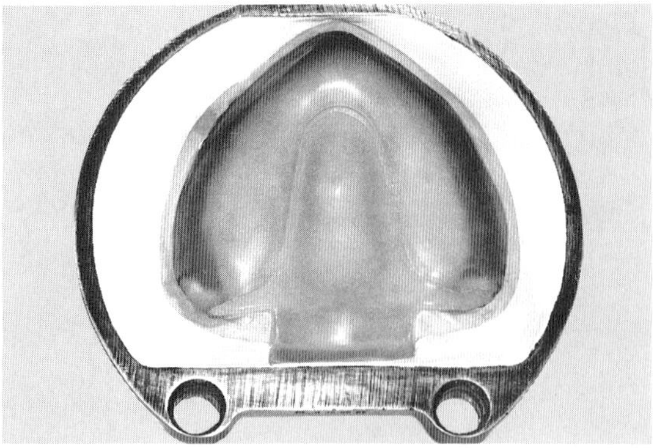

Fig. 7-10a The waxed-up maxillary base is placed into the lower member of the flask.

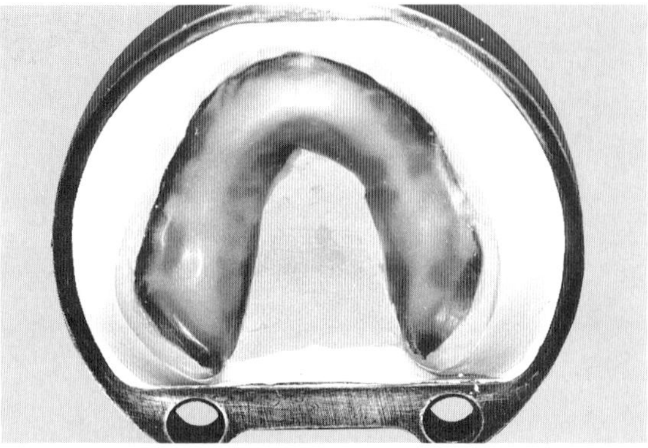

Fig. 7-10b The same procedure is performed for the mandibular base.

knife. Five minutes is adequate time to soften the wax inside the flask so that it can be opened easily. Lift off the bulk of wax with a laboratory knife or wax spatula.

5. Pour fresh boiling water over the cast and alternate with detergent* scrubs using a pastry brush. Repeat this step several times and finish with a rinse of boiling water. All soap and wax must be removed.

6. Paint one layer of tinfoil substitute† upon all stone surfaces while the cast is still warm. Allow the tinfoil substitute to dry and the cast to cool.

7. Mix approximately 48 cc of powder and 15 ml of liquid (check each manufacturer's acrylic resin for exact proportions) of the desired shade of heat-curing acrylic resin. This amount of resin is usually adequate for the average maxillary or mandibular base. Make a note of the exact shade of acrylic resin used so that there will be no question of the appropriate shade to use for the second processing. Place sufficient acrylic resin at the doughy stage into the flask and close slowly. No trial packing is necessary, because the vertical dimension of occlusion is not important at this stage. However, if there is any question at all as to whether sufficient acrylic resin has been placed in the flask, it should be trial packed.

*Ivory Liquid, Procter & Gamble, Cincinnati, Ohio.
†Al-cote, L.D. Caulk Co., Milford, Del.

8. Place the flask in the denture compress and place it in the curing tank with the water at room temperature. Heat cure the bases at 165° F for a minimum of nine hours.

9. Allow the flask to bench cool to room temperature after the curing cycle and deflask. The entire top half of the stone investment usually pries off easily if no undercuts existed in the wax-up. Remove the stone cast from inside the denture base by cutting small sections of the stone with a lathe-mounted disk.* Carefully remove each small section with a laboratory knife. Place the completed denture base in an ultrasonic cleaner, and use stone and plaster remover to remove any adhering particles of stone.

10. Remove excess flash of acrylic resin and contour the base with appropriate lathe or handpiece burs. Place a butt joint around the entire border of the denture bases using an inverted cone laboratory carbide bur (Figs. 7-11a and b). This butt joint finishing line is placed approximately 4 to 5 mm from the full extension of the denture border and should have a depth of at least 2 mm. The butt joint on the lingual surface of the mandibular base is placed higher to ensure that the base will have adequate acrylic resin for rigidity and strength.

*Damascus Separating Disks, William Dixon Co., Carlstadt, N.J.

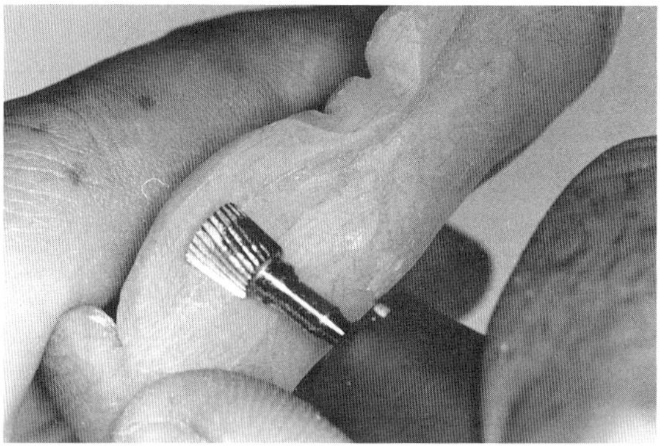

Fig. 7-11a A butt joint is placed around the entire maxillary denture base 4 mm from the full extension of the denture border.

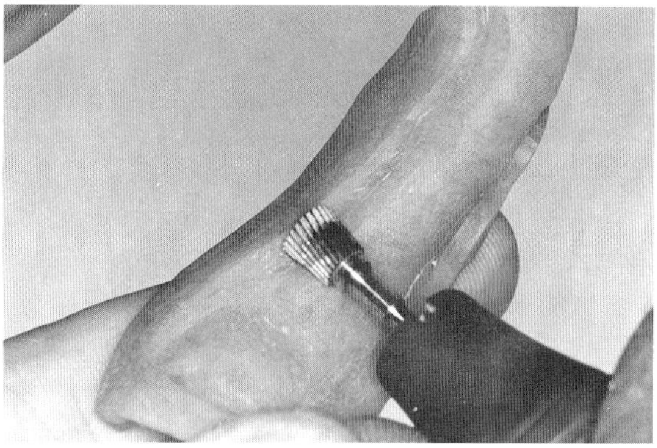

Fig. 7-11b The same procedure is performed for the mandibular base.

Roughen a small area of the acrylic resin adjacent to the butt joint with an egg-shaped carbide bur. This area is roughened so that the acrylic resin used to process the teeth will bond well to give an esthetic result. Ideally, no line of demarcation between the completed base and the second processing of acrylic resin should show.

11. Keep the completed denture base in water at all times when not working on it to prevent dimensional change caused by drying out of the acrylic resin.

Making mounting casts for completed bases

Because the casts from the final impression are destroyed to retrieve the completed denture bases, they can no longer be used for mounting on the articulator. After the completed base has been made, there is no longer a need to have the final cast because the completed base has already captured all of the detail and contour of the final impression. Because the final cast was destroyed, a new cast must be poured into the completed base so that it can be mounted upon the articulator.

The technique for fabricating mounting casts is the same for the mandibular denture as for the maxillary denture, with one exception: a wax tongue form must be added to the completed mandibular base prior to making the mounting cast.

Making the wax tongue spacer for the completed mandibular base

1. Warm a piece of baseplate wax and place the borders of the mandibular denture against the warmed wax. Using a sharp blade, follow the outline of the denture to cut a piece of wax of the proper size and shape for the tongue space.
2. Attach the cut wax to the completed base with melted baseplate wax. Make certain that wax does not touch the borders of the denture.

Preparing the completed bases and pouring casts

1. Adapt modeling material (Play-Doh*) into the tissue surface of the denture to block out all undercuts (Fig. 7-12). Place the Play-Doh up to, but not touching, the peripheral borders. Keep as much of the denture base as possible in contact with the stone. Keep the palatal and posterior palatal seal areas of the maxillary denture free of Play-Doh so that the denture will contact stone in these areas. This will help stabilize the denture upon the mounting cast and will also allow you to visually verify the full seating of the denture base in this posterior region.

* CPC Products Corp., Div. of Kenner Products, Cincinnati, Ohio.

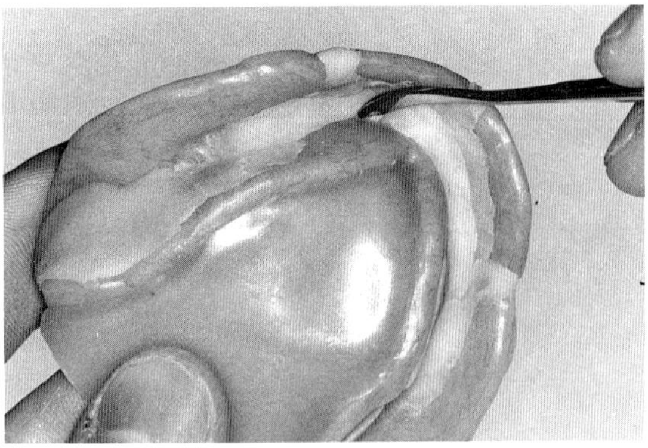

Fig. 7-12 Modeling material is adapted into the tissue surface of the denture base to block out all undercuts.

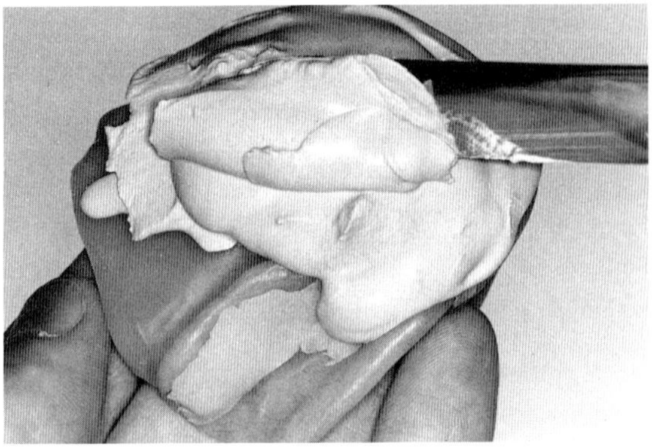

Fig. 7-13 The stone is manually vibrated into the denture base, covering all modeling material and acrylic resin surfaces.

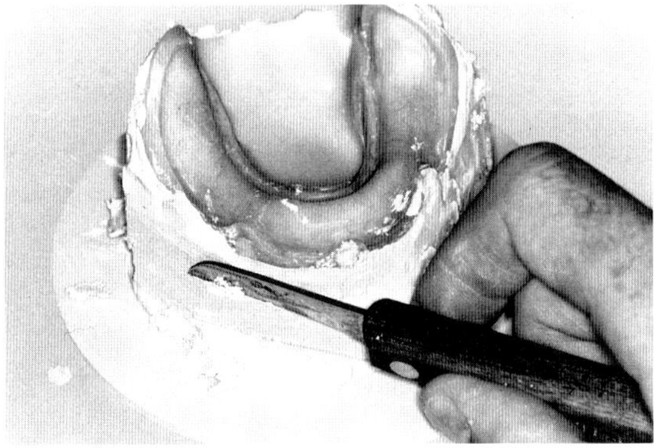

Fig. 7-14 Excess stone is cut away to expose the denture border. This is easily done if the stone is still soft.

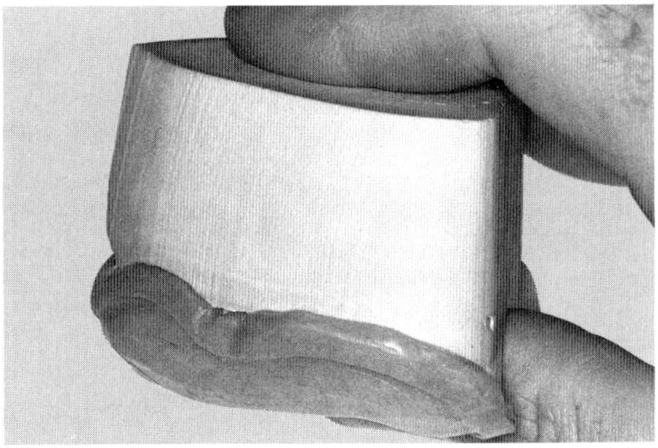

Fig. 7-15 The borders of the mounting cast are trimmed so that it is easy to visually verify the fit of the denture base to it.

2. Mix stone and slurry and manually vibrate it into the denture base, covering all the Play-Doh and the acrylic resin surfaces, including peripheral borders (Fig. 7-13).

3. Place additional stone on a tile to form a base, and invert the denture base upon the stone. Lift the stone from the base upward with a spatula toward the denture borders to ensure that all border areas are contacted by stone. Use a laboratory knife to cut excess stone away to expose the denture border. This is best accomplished before the stone gets too hard (Fig. 7-14).

4. Remove the denture base from the mounting casts by prying with a knife at the denture border. Play-Doh is an excellent material to use because it does not leave any residue on the stone or on the denture base. Any Play-Doh that is on the denture base or cast is easily removed by rinsing and brushing in tap water. In contrast, if asbestos or paper toweling is used to block out undercuts, fragments of these materials remain attached to the stone. These fragments may prevent the denture from seating completely on the mounting cast and thereby cause errors in occlusion. In addition, asbestos is a hazardous material.

Trim the base and borders of the mounting cast using laboratory knives and a model trimmer. Cut the borders of the mounting cast so that it is easy to visually verify the fit of the denture base to it (Fig. 7-15). Each time the denture base is placed upon the mounting cast, the dentist or laboratory technician can visually verify whether or not it is completely seated.

5. Notch or groove the base of the cast with a large lathe stone. This makes a definite keyway should the mounting cast separate from the articulator mounting.

Ideal requirements of a completed denture record base

To objectively evaluate the characteristics of various types of record bases (temporary and completed), some ideal requirements are presented. The ideal record base for completed dentures should:

1. Be rigid
2. Be dimensionally stable
3. Be accurately adapted to the cast, including all undercut areas, and accurately reproduce tissue detail
4. Be stable on the cast and in the mouth
5. Be as retentive in the mouth as the finished denture is expected to be
6. Be thin in appropriate areas where teeth will be set
7. Be comfortable and esthetic for the patient
8. Have the same border form as the final denture
9. Not damage the cast during its fabrication or when it is taken on and off the cast
10. Allow the dentist to evaluate the overall fit of the finished denture before proceeding to make jaw relation records and setting teeth
11. Be of reasonable cost

The completed denture base meets all of these requirements.

Advantages of completed denture bases

The advantages of using completed denture bases can be categorized into three specific areas, which are detailed as follows.

Making jaw relation records

Because the completed denture bases are as stable and retentive as the completed dentures will be, it is easy for the dentist to make the jaw relation records. It is disconcerting for the dentist and the patient when temporary bases lack retention and move around when a bite registration is being made. The added retention and stability of completed bases put the patient and dentist at ease. The lack of retention and/or stability of temporary bases can lead to errors in articulation, which are not usually evident until after the dentures are processed and inserted. The accuracy of the jaw relation records is directly related to the fit of the denture bases.

Completing (processing) the record base before making the centric relation records allows the greatest dimensional changes of the acrylic resin to occur before the final records are made, not after, as when using any temporary base. When using completed bases, it is unnecessary to remount the dentures at the insertion visit because the centric relation record was made and verified upon the completed base. Therefore, the insertion visit is a very brief visit (see chapter 14).

Because the master cast must be destroyed to retrieve a completed base, a mounting cast must be made for it. The completed bases fit accurately to the mounting casts in the same stable position every time they are placed upon them. Autopolymerizing acrylic resin temporary bases undergo dimensional changes during their set, and after being cured they may not accurately fit the master cast upon which they were made. This can lead to occlusal discrepancies, because the temporary base will fit the mouth differently than it will fit upon the cast. It is crucial to have record bases that fit accurately to the master cast.

Arranging the teeth

When using completed bases, the esthetic try-in is more precisely accomplished, primarily because the undercuts on the cast are not blocked out to fabricate it as is often done to make a temporary base. When the master cast is blocked out, the temporary base may be bulkier and may cause the lip to look unnatural. Using a completed denture base saves the dentist the time and energy of explaining to a patient that the temporary base has extra bulkiness the finished denture will not have. The esthetic appearance of a completed base at the try-in stage is the same as when the dentures are completed—there are no insertion-day surprises.

In addition, it is much easier to evaluate the esthetics and phonetics because the dentures remain in place as well as the finished dentures will. When the denture bases continually fall down or move around, as so often happens with temporary bases, one cannot properly or easily evaluate tooth position. Denture adhesives can make the patient feel uncomfortable. The patient becomes concerned as to whether the finished denture is going to fall out of his mouth as readily as the temporary bases do. The use of adhesives also gives the patient false security as to the steadfastness of the final denture, and the adhesive is a nuisance to clean from the patient's mouth. During the try-in of the teeth, the patient may be concerned about how the final dentures will fit and not concentrate upon the appearance of the teeth.

Another advantage of using a completed denture base is that the patient may take home the wax try-in stage of the completed denture base to more critically evaluate the trial denture (see chapter 11). This allows the patient and friends or family to comment upon the final arrangement of the teeth before the final processing.

Evaluating the fit

The dentist has the opportunity to evaluate the overall fit (retention and stability) of the finished denture prior to making jaw relation records and certainly before making any commitment to the patient to finish the dentures. Overextensions or pressure areas on the denture bases can be adjusted before any jaw relation records are made. If the retention and/or the stability is not adequate, the dentist may elect to make corrections before proceeding with the treatment.

References

1. Brewer, A.A. Prosthodontic research in progress at the School of Aerospace Medicine. J. Prosthet. Dent. 13(13):49, 1963.
2. Graser, G.N. Completed bases for removable dentures. J. Prosthet. Dent. 39:232, 1978.
3. Vig, R.G. Method of reducing the shifting of teeth in denture processing. J. Prosthet. Dent. 33:80–84, 1975.

The accuracy of a centric jaw relation record is directly related to the stability, retention, and fit of the record bases it is made upon. Regardless of the method, precision, or clinical skill employed to obtain this record, any difference between the bases on which the record is obtained and the completed denture will invalidate the record. Ideally, the denture base should be completed before the jaw relation records are made.

Allen Brewer
(Personal communication)

Chapter 8

Maxillomandibular Relations: Articulators, Vertical Dimension, and Centric Jaw Relation

Articulators

Dentists have over 300 different articulators to choose from, and their selection continues to be a fashionable topic to discuss. Most removable prostheses are fabricated outside of the dental office in a commercial dental laboratory. This "remote" place of fabrication makes it necessary for the dentist to provide the laboratory technicians with enough information and jaw relation records to use the selected articulator properly. The quality of the occlusion developed by the dentist and/or laboratory technician depends upon the precision of the jaw relation records, the capabilities of the articulator being used, and the skill of the dentist and laboratory technician.

Many dentists argue that the best articulator is the patient's mouth, because that is where the prosthesis ends up and that is where it "has to be adjusted anyway." Contrary to that belief, others state that the articulator is the best means of developing the occlusal scheme because *(1)* visibility is best outside of the mouth where not influenced by intraoral factors such as saliva, poor light, and patient cooperation, *(2)* the patient's closure and eccentric movements can be repeatedly controlled, and *(3)* time spent doing intraoral adjustment is greatly minimized, saving both the dentist and patient frustrating moments. An articulator is used to relate casts to one another so as to mechanically simulate the static and functional positions of the mandible. By using the appropriate articulator, each laboratory and clinical step in the development of the occlusion can be made easier, better, and more enjoyable.

Selecting the appropriate articulator

The development of articulatory instruments has taken two major paths. The first group of researchers developed geometric theories of occlusion. This school was led by Bonwill[1] in the mid-19th century and Monson[2] in the early 20th century. Bonwill postulated that the distance between the mandibular condyles and the mandibular symphysis formed an equilateral 4-inch triangle, and he designed an articulator based upon that theory. Monson postulated that mandibular motion occurred around a 4-inch sphere, and he also developed an articulator that allowed artificial teeth to be set to contact the surface of his 4-inch sphere. The second group of researchers designed articulators to simulate the various movements made by the temporomandibular joint. Hundreds of such articulators have been developed, some of which are capable of considerable acrobatics in their attempts to mechanically simulate the movement of the mandible.

Articulators are most commonly classified according to how closely they mimic centric and eccentric mandibular movements. The articulators that are the least adjustable are called *simple* or *hinge* articulators because they have very limited capabilities for simulating eccentric mandibular positions. The articulators that mimic mandibular motion to the greatest degree are called *fully adjustable* articulators. *Semiadjustable* articulators fall between the two and generally simulate the movements of the mandible fairly closely.

Articulators are also described with regard to whether their "condyles" are on the instrument's

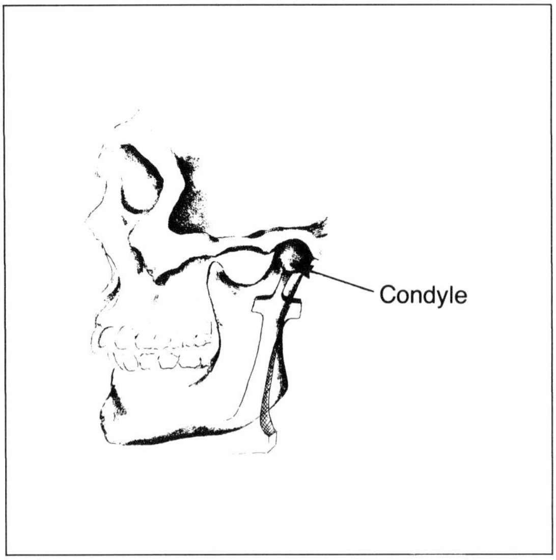

Fig. 8-1a On an arcon articulator, the condyle is part of the mandibular member of the instrument.

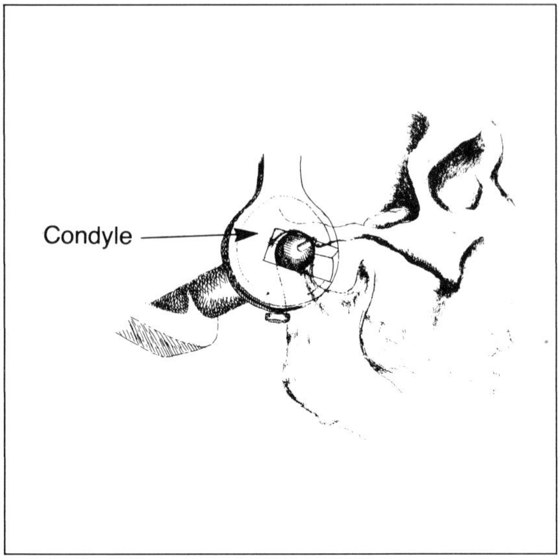

Fig. 8-1b On a nonarcon articulator, the condyle is part of the maxillary member of the articulator.

"maxilla" (upper member) or "mandible" (lower member). On an *arcon* articulator, the condyle is part of the mandibular member of the instrument to simulate the human state (Fig. 8-1a). On a *nonarcon* articulator, the condyle is part of the maxillary member of the instrument—just the opposite of how the temporomandibular joint is arranged (Fig. 8-1b).

On an arcon articulator, the controlling mechanism (the part that determines how the articulator will move) is attached to the maxillary member. On a nonarcon articulator, the controlling mechanism is attached to the mandibular member. The advantage of using an arcon articulator is that the condylar settings remain the same when the vertical dimension of occlusion is changed. A nonarcon articulator's condylar settings change when the vertical dimension is altered.

Another important distinction between articulators is whether they are *tracking* or *nontracking*. The tracking instruments have a rigid, totally boxed-in slot in which the condylar ball moves (Fig. 8-2). The nontracking instruments are not totally boxed in, so that the maxillary member of the articulator can be removed from the mandibular member (Fig. 8-3). Some articulators are programmed or set to move in *rectilinear* (straight) paths (Fig. 8-4), whereas others are programmed or set to move in *curvilinear* (curved) paths (Fig. 8-5). The mandible itself generally moves in curvilinear paths, and articulators that simulate these paths are considered to be more adjustable.

Many think that the occlusion developed in a complete denture is relatively unimportant because the dentures rest upon soft tissues with no "fixed" support and therefore move in function. However, the occlusion developed in complete dentures can also be thought of as being very important because the better the occlusion, the more stable and comfortable the dentures will be.

The criteria for selecting an articulator for removable prosthodontics will now be discussed. The dentist should determine the occlusal requirements of each patient and then select an instrument that will best help meet them.

1. *The articulator should be rigid and maintain all centric and eccentric positions.* The rigidity of the instrument, the quality of the materials used to make it, and its workmanship will determine whether the articulator will hold the relationships that were programmed into it. When an articulator is made of weak materials or is machined poorly, a significant amount of play can occur. A once-

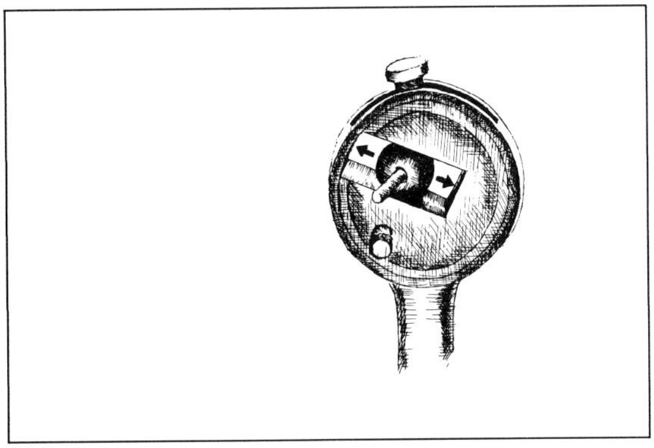

Fig. 8-2 A tracking instrument has a rigid, totally boxed-in slot in which the condylar ball moves.

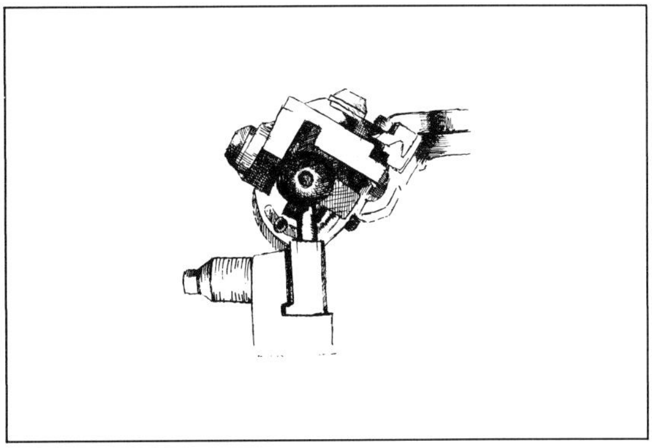

Fig. 8-3 On a nontracking instrument, the condylar ball is not totally boxed in.

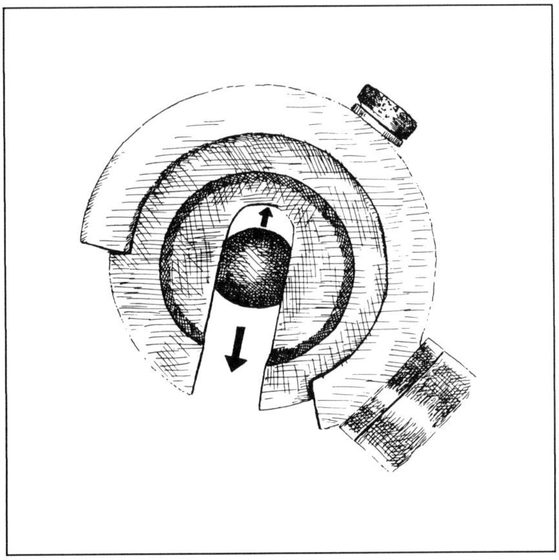

Fig. 8-4 Rectilinear instruments move in straight lines.

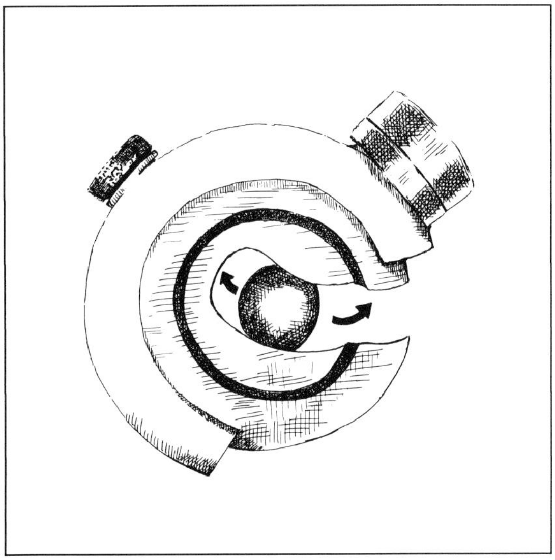

Fig. 8-5 Curvilinear instruments move in curved paths.

accurate mounting is no longer accurate when the articulator does not hold its position.

2. *The articulator should have an incisal guide pin and an adjustable guide table.* The pin itself is important in maintaining the vertical relationship of the teeth. The adjustable guide table is used as a controlling factor as denture teeth are set up. The incisal guide pin should touch the guide table in each lateral and protrusive movement to ensure that the selected incisal guidance is maintained and to ensure against displacement of previously set teeth. As the denture teeth are set up, one by one, the guide pin should be watched to make certain that it remains upon the table. The incisal guide pin and table are also significant in that they simulate the end controlling factors of incisal guidance while the anterior teeth are being set up.

3. *The articulator should have an adjustable condylar inclination and be able to accept a protrusive record to set it.* If the movement of the articulator between the centric jaw relation and

protrusive position is rectilinear (straight), we only know where the patient will be positioned in the centric jaw relation and protrusive positions. The complication arises in that we do not know the precise patient mandibular position as the articulator is moved between each of these points. The rectilinear instrument selects an "average" movement, while a fully adjustable instrument can accurately track the patient's protrusive movement.

4. *The articulator should accept an arbitrary face-bow transfer.* The maxillary cast is related to the arbitrary horizontal axis of rotation through the use of the face-bow and then mounted upon the articulator. The mandibular cast is later mounted to the maxillary cast with a centric jaw relation record; therefore, the mandibular cast is then related to the horizontal axis of rotation. An arbitrary face-bow record reduces the occlusal discrepancy that can occur if the vertical dimension of occlusion is altered.

5. *The articulator should have an adjustable Bennett angle and an average Bennett movement programmed into it.* Hanau suggests the use of the following formula to set the Bennett angle on the Hanau articulator[3]:

$$\text{Bennett angle} = \frac{\text{condylar inclination}}{8} + 12$$

This formula has absolutely no scientific basis. When using this formula, a difference in the condylar inclination of 20° (from 10° to 30°) changes the product of the formula only 2.5° (from 13.25° to 15.75°). Gysi found that the average Bennett angle was approximately 15°.[4] This was the basis behind the development of the Hanau formula. No matter what value is determined for the condylar inclination, the Bennett angle will be approximately 15°. Therefore, it is reasonable to arbitrarily set the Bennett angle at 15° and leave it there. The greater the Bennett angle, the flatter the cusps will be.

The Bennett angle of nontracking articulators (Denar,* Whip Mix†) can be set by making lateral checkbite records. A tracking articulator such as the Hanau H2 will not accept lateral checkbites to set the Bennett angle. The amount of Bennett movement that is achieved on the Hanau H2* articulator is a function of the degree of Bennett angle set. If the Bennett angle were set at 0°, there would be no Bennett movement. The Bennett movement as machined into the instrument is dependent upon the balancing condylar motion. When a 0° Bennett angle is set, the working condyle rotates without any lateral shift. Try this on a Hanau articulator.

Many describe the Hanau H2 as the workhorse for removable prosthodontics. However, although the illustrations and photographs in this book show the Hanau H2, they are not meant to be an exclusive endorsement of the articulator. Other semi-adjustable instruments work equally well.

*Denar Mark II, Denar Corp., Anaheim, Calif.
†Whip Mix Model 8500, Whip Mix Corp., Louisville, Ky.

The face-bow record

1. Make a wax occlusion rim upon the completed maxillary base. Contour the rim to the maxillary arch form so that it is 22 mm long, from the height of the labial flange in the canine region to the incisal edge of the wax rim. Progressively shorten the occlusal height of the rim posteriorly to simulate the anticipated plane of occlusion. The rim should be thinner (labially-palatally) in the anterior region than in the posterior region to simulate the thickness of the teeth in each region.

2. Attach the face-bow bite fork to the maxillary rim by warming the fork under a flame and then immediately inserting it through the wax rim. Hold the fork steadily in place until the wax is hardened, or immerse it in cold water. The fork should be centered in the wax rim so that the face-bow record can be made comfortably, without pushing too hard upon the lip. To save chair time, steps 1 and 2 can be done before the patient's scheduled appointment.

3. Place a thin layer of pressure-indicating material† inside of both completed bases using the supplied brush (Fig. 8-6). Check the overall fit of the completed bases before any records are made

*Hanau Model 96 H2, Teledyne Hanau Co., Buffalo, N.Y.
†Pressure Indicating Paste, Mizzy Co., Clifton Forge, Va.

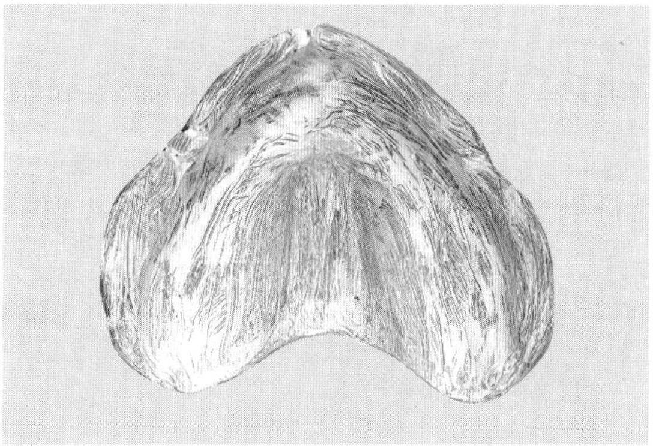

Fig. 8-6 A thin layer of pressure-indicating material is applied inside the completed base. A bristle brush is used so that brush marks are evident upon the entire surface.

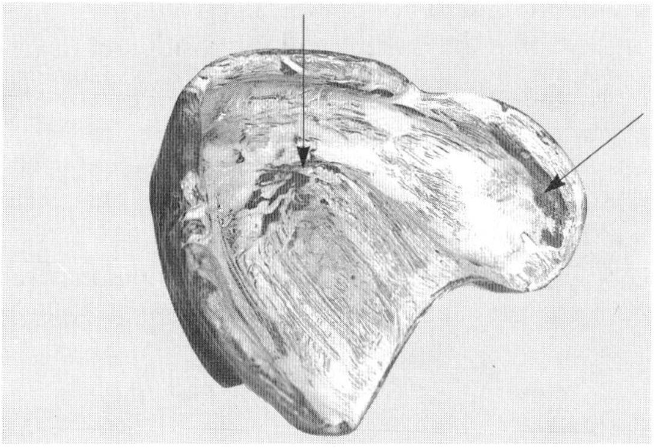

Fig. 8-7 The completed bases with pressure-indicating material are inserted in the patient's mouth and removed to check for obvious pressure areas *(arrows)*.

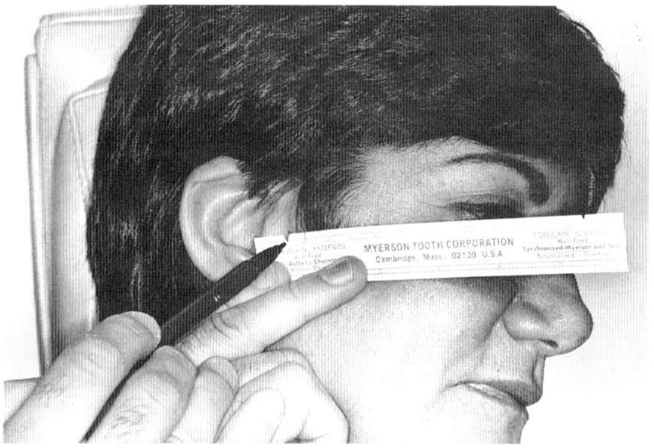

Fig. 8-8 Beyron's arbitrary hinge axis point is marked on the patient's face.

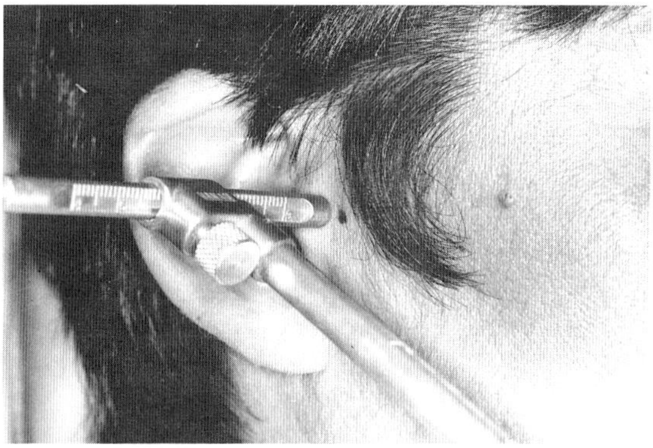

Fig. 8-9 The face-bow is adjusted so that the condylar axis arms touch the marked Beyron's points at the same number on the indexed scale.

(Fig. 8-7). The fitting of the completed bases at this time is done mainly to ensure that the patient will be comfortable and to correct for any processing changes *before* the jaw relation records are made. As mentioned in chapter 7, it is at this time that the overall stability and retention can be evaluated. If the bases do not fit appropriately or as expected, a decision must be made as to whether to modify the bases or make another impression.

4. Locate and mark Beyron's arbitrary hinge axis point on the patient's skin (Fig. 8-8). Beyron's point is located 13 mm from the most posterior portion of the tragus of the ear on a line with the outer canthus of the eye.

5. Insert the completed maxillary record base with the attached bite fork in the patient's mouth. Position the face-bow apparatus to fit into the bite fork arm, and then adjust the side axis arms so that they are equidistant from the axis points on the face when the axis arms just touch the marked points (Fig. 8-9). Tighten the connection of the fork to the face-bow itself. Loosen the axis arms bilaterally, and check to see that each arm aligns with Beyron's point. Replace the axis arm into contact with the skin and observe the number on the indexed scale. If the arms do not touch the skin at the same number, either *(1)* repeat step 5, or *(2)* write the numbers that the axis rods touch Beyron's

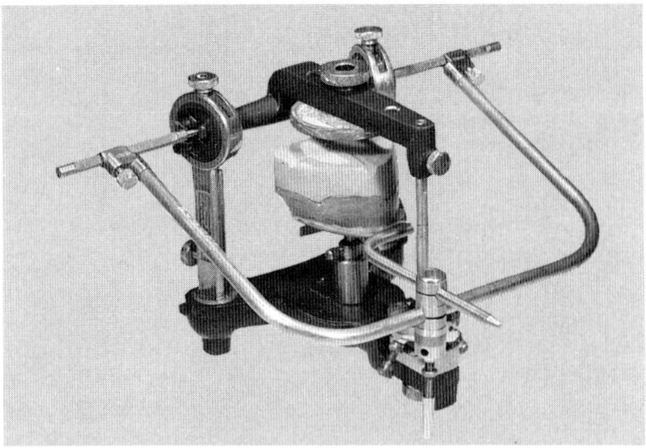

Fig. 8-10 The incisal edge of the maxillary occlusion rim is positioned level with the line on the incisal guide pin.

point on a piece of paper. Take an average between these two figures and adjust the face-bow assembly to touch the articulator condylar axis rods using the average numerical ratio.

6. Remove the face-bow from the patient and attach it to the articulator condylar rods. If the condylar axis arms of the face-bow touched the face with equal bilateral values, then attach the face-bow to the articulator with the arms equal. If the condylar axis arms of the face-bow touched the face with unequal values, then attach the arms to the articulator with the same ratio of numbers.

7. Adjust the anterior height of the maxillary occlusion rim by moving the face-bow up and down so that the incisal edge of the maxillary occlusion rim is level with the line on the incisal guide pin (Fig. 8-10).

8. Place the mounting cast in the processed maxillary base and mount it on the articulator with stone and slurry. The mounting cast should be soaked for 15 minutes in supersaturated calcium sulfate solution to achieve a better bond to the mounting stone.

9. Remove the bite fork from the occlusion rim by warming the handle of the bite fork directly under the flame. The heat will be conducted to the fork, which is embedded in the wax rim. The wax will melt and make removal of the fork easy. Readapt wax to the rim to fill in the voids left by the fork.

Vertical dimension and centric jaw relation

Establishing the correct maxillomandibular relationships can be one of the most perplexing aspects of prosthodontics, especially when treating the complete denture patient. A centric jaw relation record is made at a particular vertical dimension of occlusion; therefore, the record is made with the mandible in a specific three-dimensional relationship to the maxilla. When a few teeth remain in occlusion prior to the fabrication of complete dentures, they can provide valuable insight to establish the appropriate vertical dimension of occlusion and occlusal positions. Diagnostic casts are a must before the teeth are extracted.

Although many methods for determining maxillomandibular relationships have been suggested, no one technique has been demonstrated to be the best. Whatever techniques are used, meticulous care should be used to verify that the relationships are correct.

Vertical dimension

The *vertical dimension of the face* refers to the facial height that exists between two arbitrarily selected points, one in the mandible and the other in the maxilla (or upper part of the face) (Fig. 8-11). The *vertical dimension of occlusion* refers to the face height that exists when the teeth are in occlusion. The *vertical dimension of rest* (or the *clinical rest position*[5]) has been defined as the habitual postural position of the mandible when the patient is resting comfortably in an upright position and the condyles are in a neutral, unstrained position in the glenoid fossa.[6] The *interocclusal distance* or *freeway space* is defined as that space that exists between the teeth when the mandible is in the clinical rest position (Fig. 8-12).

Many ideas have been proposed regarding the lifelong stability of a person's vertical jaw relations. Thompson suggested that the mandible assumes its final positional relationship to the head by the third month of life and does not change after that point.[7] Basically, he believed that the clinical rest position is constant throughout life, from birth to death.

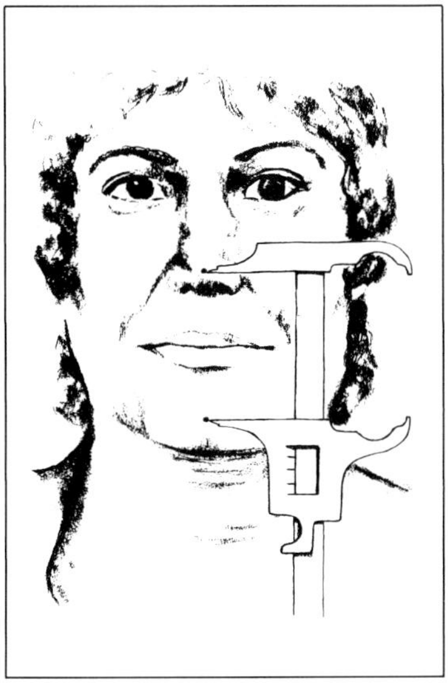

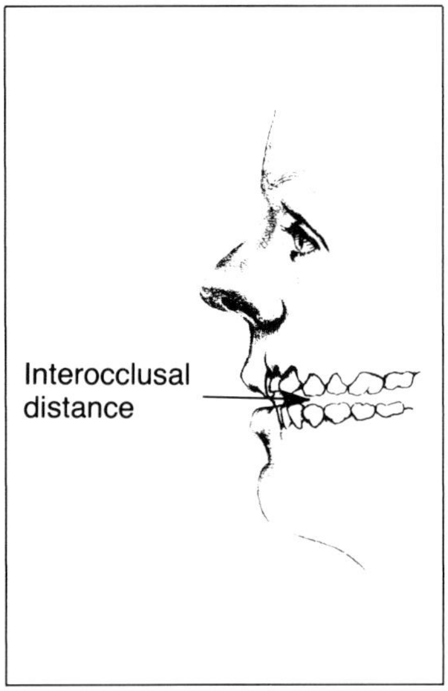

Fig. 8-11 *(left)* One point is located in the mandible and the other in the maxilla (or upper face). The distance between these two points, as measured with a caliper, is the vertical dimension.

Fig. 8-12 *(right)* Clinical rest position showing the available interocclusal distance.

Those who shared his view believed that the clinical rest position was unaffected by the eruption of or loss of teeth. More current research has shown that the rest position is not constant. Atwood studied 42 patients before and after the extraction of teeth that maintained the vertical dimension of occlusion.[5] Complete dentures were then fabricated. The clinical rest position was found to vary within a single patient visit, between visits, and with and without the dentures in the mouth. Sometimes large variations in the clinical rest position existed pre- and postextraction. Of the 42 patients, 11 showed an increase in the resting vertical dimension following the extraction of the teeth, 9 remained at basically the same clinical rest position, and 22 showed a decrease. Tallgren stated that because of the inconsistency and variability of the clinical rest position, it is an unreliable reference point for establishing the vertical dimension of occlusion.[8]

Several other methods are used to determine the vertical dimension of occlusion. These include phonetics, swallowing, bite force, patient preference, and esthetics. Each method has its indications for use and each is useful in evaluating the vertical dimension of occlusion. Clinical experience is necessary when determining the correct vertical dimension, because no one method has been proven best.

The techniques described in this book combine intraoral measurements, clinical rest position, phonetics, and esthetics. The initial, tentative vertical dimension of occlusion is selected based upon some average measurements. This assessment is made prior to making the centric jaw relation record; it is later reassessed using phonetics and esthetics. The most significant evaluation of the vertical dimension of occlusion comes when the teeth are set up and tried in the patient's mouth. Evaluating the vertical dimension of occlusion at the wax rim stage is most difficult and at best tentative. It is only after all of the teeth have been set that a real sense of the appropriate vertical dimension of occlusion can be obtained.

McGrane was the first to write about the use of an average value in determining the occlusal dimension.[9] He measured hundreds of casts and found that the distance between the maxillary and mandibular labial frena averaged 40 mm. The technique to be described also uses a 40-mm measurement, but this distance is measured from the periphery of the denture flanges in the regions of the maxillary and mandibular canines (Fig. 8-13). Graser, Plekavich, and Espeland have shown that the natural dentition has a mean value of 37.7 mm (with the teeth in centric occlusion) when the depth of the labial sulcus is measured from the maxilla to the mandible in the region of the canines[10]:

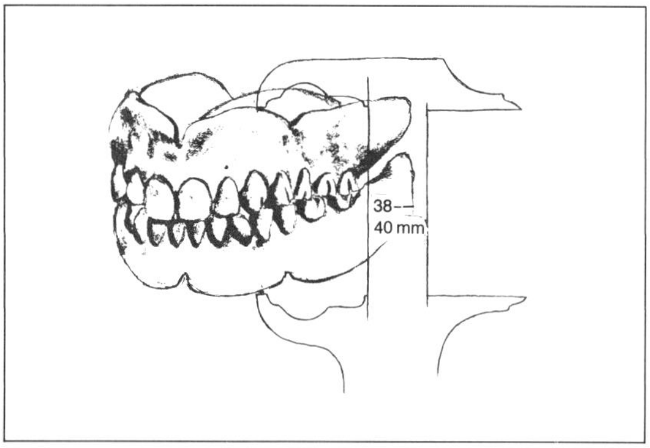

Fig. 8-13 For complete dentures, a measurement is made from the height of the denture borders in the canine regions of the maxillary and mandibular dentures.

Figs. 8-14a and b As a preliminary measure, the denture teeth are set using average values.

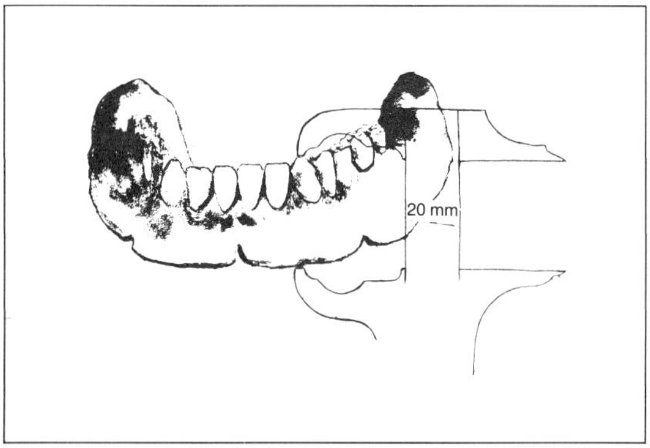

Fig. 8-14a

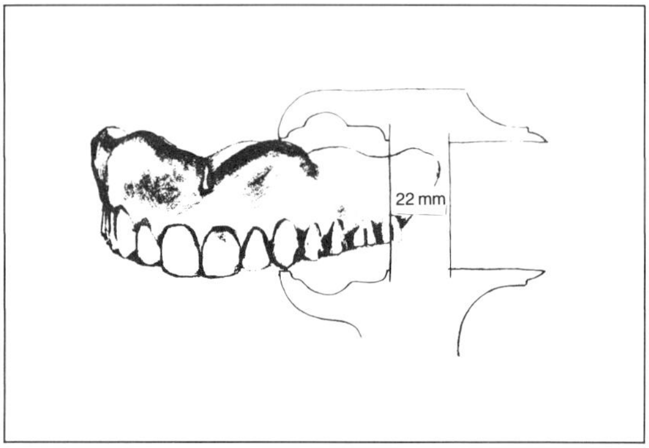

Fig. 8-14b

The use of average value measurements for the replacement of missing anterior teeth has been reported but not documented. The purpose of this study is to use anthropometric measurements and establish mean values for the position of anterior central incisors and cuspids. The vertical dimension of occlusion will be determined by measuring from maxillary to mandibular labial sulci.

One hundred and twenty-three subjects between 22 and 60 years of age were used to record the anterior tooth position and labial sulcus anatomy. Polyvinylsiloxane impression material was injected into the anterior part of the mouth from cuspid to cuspid while the teeth were in centric occlusion and the lips in a natural repose. The resultant impression was measured from the labial sulci to the center of the incisal edges of both the maxillary and mandibular central incisors and cuspids. The total distance from labial sulcus (maxillae) to labial sulcus (mandible) in the region of the central incisors and cuspids was also recorded. Correlations were made with the subject's height, sex, and age.

The mean distance (mm) from the mucolabial reflection to the center of the maxillary central incisor edge was 20.1 Right and 20.2 Left, and for the cuspid, 21.2 R, 21.4 L. For the mandible, the measurements from the mucolabial fold to the central incisors were 16.7 R, 16.5 L and 19.4 R, 19.2 L for the cuspid. The mean total distance from sulcus to sulcus in the region of the central incisors was 33.5 R and 33.5 L, while for the cuspids it was 37.7 R and 37.7 L.

A positive relationship between the subject's height and the distance from sulcus to sulcus in the region of the central incisors and canines was found to be statistically significant ($p < 0.10$). The differences between means for males and females could largely be explained by differences in height. No statistically significant difference could be found for age.

The results of Graser, Plekavich, and Espeland's study can be applied to the edentulous patient.

Since edentulous impression procedures usually displace the mucolabial sulcus, an additional 2 to 3 mm may be added to the natural dentition figures. Therefore, the 40-mm figure is a good place to start. Use an average measurement of 20 mm for the mandible and 22 mm for the maxilla as measured from the tip of the canine to the height of the flange (Figs. 8-14a and b). It must be kept in mind that these are average values and may have to be altered, depending upon the patient being treated.

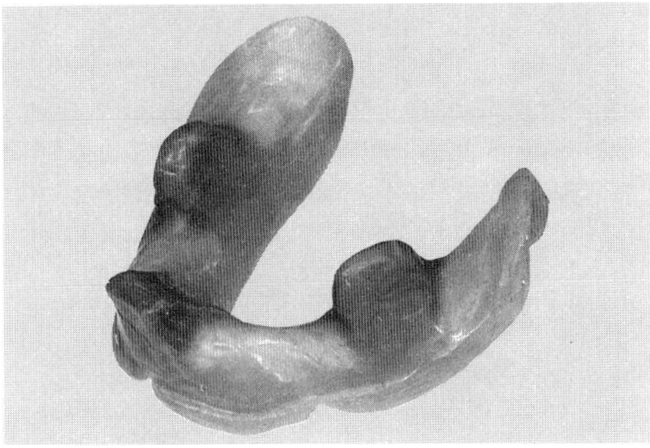

Fig. 8-15 Three wax blocks approximately 18 to 20 mm high are placed on the completed mandibular base.

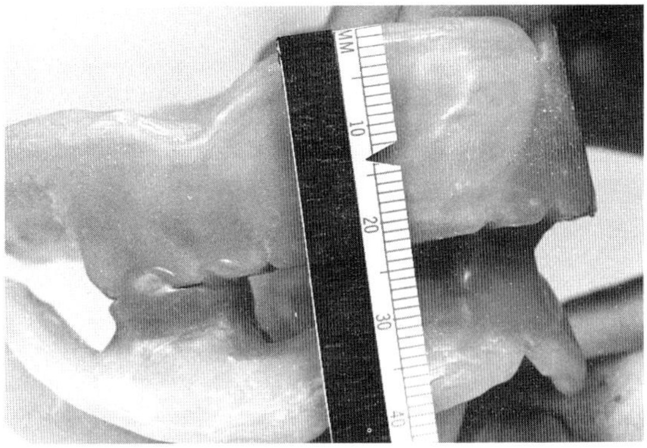

Fig. 8-16 Each wax-up should touch the maxillary rim, and a measurement of the distance between the denture border extensions in the canine areas should be made.

Technique for initial assessment of vertical dimension of occlusion

1. Place three small baseplate wax nubs (approximately 18 to 20 mm high) on the completed mandibular base—one in the anterior region and two in the molar regions (Fig. 8-15). Flow some baseplate wax under the wax blocks and around their periphery to secure them to the baseplate. Adjust the anterior wax block to be about 18 mm from the labial flange as measured from the flange periphery in the labial frenum area. Adjust the molar-positioned blocks to be approximately one half to two thirds the height of the retromolar pad.

2. Insert the maxillary and mandibular record bases in the patient's mouth while the wax blocks are still soft, and guide the patient to close into the centric jaw relation position. Remove both denture bases from the mouth. Be sure that the wax blocks have contacted the maxillary occlusion rim, and measure the distance between the canine flange areas (Fig. 8-16). If the measurement is approximately 37 to 40 mm, reinsert the bases in the mouth and use some phonetic tests. Instruct the patient to count from 50 to 60, and pay particular attention to the sibilant ("s") sounds. During articulation of the "s" sound, the mandibular anterior teeth move downward and forward to within approximately 1 mm of the incisal edges of the maxillary anterior teeth. Assess the distance between the wax blocks and maxillary occlusion rim when the "s" sound is made. (For complete details on using phonetics in evaluating the vertical dimension, see chapter 11—phonetics, as a test of vertical dimension, is best used and understood when teeth are set up.) The clinical rest position also can be evaluated at this stage to see that there is adequate interocclusal distance. Make a centric jaw relation record at this tentative vertical dimension of occlusion.

Centric jaw relation and centric occlusion

There is controversy about which jaw relation position to use—centric jaw relation or centric occlusion. According to *The Glossary of Prosthodontic Terms*, *centric jaw relation* is defined as *(1)* the jaw relation when the condyles are in the most posterior, unstrained position in the glenoid fossae at any given degree of jaw separation from which lateral movement can be made; *(2)* the most posterior relation of the mandible to the maxillae at the established vertical dimension; *(3)* the relation of the mandible to the maxillae when the condyles are in their most posterior position in the glenoid fossae from which unstrained lateral movements can be made at the occluding vertical dimension normal for the individual.[6]

Centric jaw relation is a condylar-determined position, not a tooth-determined position. Centric jaw relation records are made without the influ-

Table 8-1 Investigations of centric jaw relation (CJR)–centric occlusion (CO) discrepancies*

Dentulous subjects	Discrepancy between CJR–CO_{ap}†	Range CJR–CO_{ap}	Discrepancy between CJR–CO_{ml}‡	Range CJR–CO_{ml}
Posselt (1952)[11]	1.25§	---	---	---
Temple (1959)[12]	.35	.00–.80	.20	---
Kydd and Sander (1961)[13]	.87	.20–1.80	---	---
Beyron (1964)[14]	1.15	.00–2.00	---	---
Ingervall (1964)[15]	.89	.30–2.00	.16	.00–.60
Hodge and Mahan (1967)[16]	.44	---	.01	---
Helkimo et al. (1971)[17]	1.65	---	---	---
Agerberg (1971)[18]	1.04	---	---	---

*Although these data are listed in tabular form, comparisons cannot be drawn because experiments were done under different conditions and with different interpretations and analyses.
†ap = anterior-posterior discrepancy.
‡ml = medial-lateral discrepancy.
§All measurements in millimeters.

ences of tooth contacts. Centric jaw relation position is dependent upon the operator guiding the patient's mandible into this position. When the centric jaw relation position is used, the vertical dimension of occlusion can be altered on the articulator without fear of changing tooth positions, assuming that the true hinge axis was located and transferred to the articulator using a face-bow. An arbitrary face-bow record will minimize the potential errors if the vertical dimension of occlusion is altered. Centric jaw relation records eliminate retrusive considerations in the occlusal scheme. All patient function will take place anterior or lateral to centric jaw relation.

Centric occlusion, on the other hand, is defined as the maximum intercuspation of the dentition. It is a tooth contact–determined position, not a condylar-determined position. The patient's free, habitual, and *unguided* closure determines the centric occlusion position. An operator does not guide the patient's mandible into this position as with centric jaw relation records. When a patient opens or closes into a habitual centric occlusion, there is no pure rotation about a horizontal axis. The mandible translates as well as rotates without a single common center. Therefore, it is impossible to make centric occlusion records at an increased vertical dimension using a recording medium that separates the teeth. In this situation, after removal of the recording medium, the teeth on the casts would come together in an incorrect position because the articulator axle only rotates, while the mandible would translate and rotate to closure. Therefore, use of interocclusal records at other than the correct vertical dimension is not an accurate method for mounting casts in a centric occlusion position.

Previous studies on *dentulous* subjects have shown that there is usually a discrepancy between a patient's centric jaw relation position and centric occlusion position (Table 8-1).[11–18]

In a study of 25 *edentulous* patients, Graser has shown that the discrepancy between centric jaw relation and centric occlusion was 1.03 mm anteroposteriorly and 0.24 mm mediolaterally.[19] Of the subjects, 80% had at least a 0.5-mm discrepancy. The centric occlusion position was significantly reproducible. The difference between the recordings anteroposteriorly was only 0.10 mm. There was no difference between mean recordings of the centric occlusion position mediolaterally. The difference between recordings anteroposteriorly for the centric jaw relation position was 0.05 mm, and there was no mediolateral difference.

In the second part of this study, Graser constructed duplicate mandibular dentures for six edentulous patients.[20] One denture was fabricated to the centric jaw relation position, the other to the centric occlusion position. Although no definite preference was established for either denture, two patients did prefer the centric jaw relation position denture for esthetic reasons, and one patient preferred the centric occlusion denture. Graser concluded that the centric occlusion position can be clinically acceptable for the intercuspation of artificial teeth for complete dentures.

The clinical significance of Graser's studies is twofold. First, even if the centric jaw relation position is located accurately, almost all patients will have a centric occlusion position anterior and lateral to it, which points out the importance of being able to balance the occlusion in protrusion. Second, because each of the six patients in the second part of Graser's study could function with either the centric jaw relation or the centric occlusion denture, it appears that the horizontal component of the centric position is not as critical as the vertical component. It is most important that both the right and left sides of the denture contact at the same time upon closure.

Methods of recording the centric jaw relation position can be broadly classified as *static*, *graphic*, or *functional*. Static records include the direct intraoral checkbite method using a material (wax, compound, zinc oxide and eugenol, or some other) interposed between the occlusion rims. Graphic records make use of intraoral or extraoral tracing devices and a central bearing point secured to the record bases. Functional records are made by using pantographic tracers or metal studs that cut tracings into an opposing material such as wax. Any of these methods can be used to make centric records with completed bases. In fact, because of the stability and retention of completed bases, they would increase the accuracy of the record. The most important factor is that no matter how the recordings are made, they must later be verified as correct.

The method to be described in this chapter for recording centric jaw relation is classified as a static method. It is recommended because it has been found to be practical and to yield very reproducible results. More importantly, the Centric Check Point* method for verifying the accuracy of the centric jaw relation records will be detailed. The Centric Check Points were developed to verify the centric jaw relation record no matter which method was used to record it. The centric occlusion position for each patient will also be visualized using checkpoints. Mounting the casts using the centric occlusion position is sometimes required. Indications for centric occlusion mounting will be discussed in this chapter.

Technique for making the centric jaw relation record

1. Cut small V-shaped grooves (3 mm deep) into the maxillary occlusion rim in the areas where the lower wax blocks touch it. Lightly rub petroleum jelly over these areas, and insert the maxillary base in the mouth.
2. Uniformly soften the wax nubs at their tops, and insert the mandibular base in the mouth. The less wax that is softened, the smaller the chance of error caused by shrinkage of the wax as it cools.
3. Secure the completed mandibular base with your forefinger, and reflect the upper lip with your middle fingers (Fig. 8-17). Use your middle fingers to stabilize the maxillary base at the same time. Place your thumbs upon the patient's chin to support and help guide the mandible. The purpose of this bilateral hand position technique is to stabilize the bases, reflect the lips to improve visibility, and to gently guide the mandible with even bilateral control.
4. Guide the patient's mandible to make the centric jaw relation record. When using wax, the mandible can be opened and closed into the wax record while the wax is still soft to verify accuracy. When using stone or Z0E as a recording medium, the patient and the bases must be held absolutely still until the material sets. Regardless of which material is used, the record should be checked intraorally before mounting on the articulator. Make certain that no parts of the record bases themselves are in contact in the retromolar pad–maxillary tuberosity region (Figs. 8-18a and b). This contact

*Teledyne Hanau Co., Buffalo, N.Y.

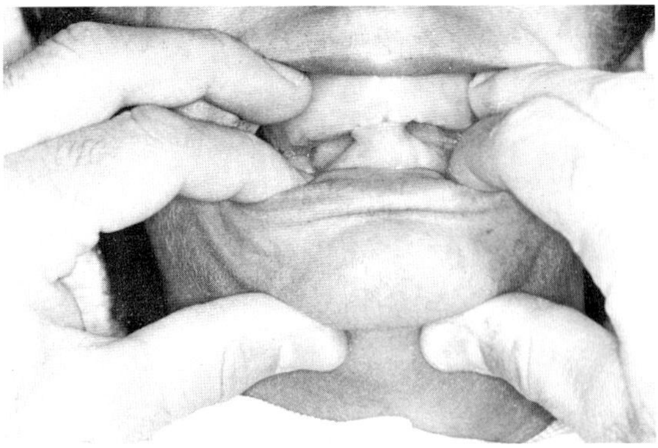

Fig. 8-17 The mandibular base is held in position with the forefinger while the middle fingers reflect the lip and stabilize the maxillary base.

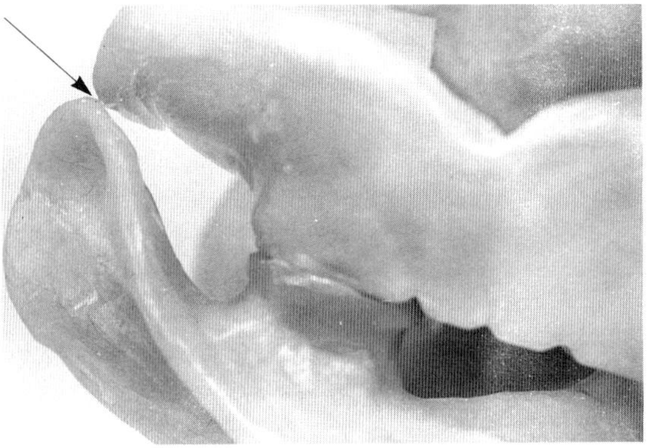

Fig. 8-18a Before mounting the bases, make certain that the record bases themselves are not in contact in the retromolar pad–maxillary tuberosity region. Here they are touching *(arrow)*.

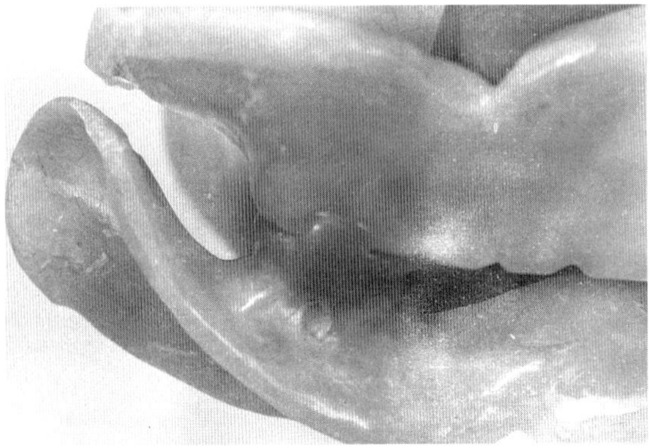

Fig. 8-18b Acrylic resin has been reduced to provide adequate clearance.

may cause an error when the record is made because it is likely to make the bases shift. The bases should be adjusted so that no contact exists, and a new record made.

5. Secure the maxillary and mandibular bases to the mounting casts with sticky wax, and then secure the wax blocks to the maxillary occlusion rim in the same manner. Use stone and slurry to mount the completed mandibular base. As soon as the stone has set, take the record bases off of the mounting casts and remove the maxillary occlusion rim and the mandibular wax blocks in preparation for using the Centric Check Points. An apparently accurate centric jaw relation record has been made and transferred to the articulator. However, an error could have occurred when the record was made or when the record was transferred and mounted on the articulator.

Centric jaw relation verification

Centric Check Points, as developed by Brewer,[21] are used to verify that a correct centric record was made and that the record was mounted correctly on the articulator. When Centric Check Points are used in conjunction with completed bases, the need for remounting the dentures at the time of insertion is eliminated. Successful use of this technique for centric jaw relation record verification is based on the use of stable, retentive, and comfortable bases.

Technique for using checkpoints

1. Assemble the checkpoints for use; a complete set consists of three short points, three medium points, three long points, three small cups, three large cups, and one wrench. Screw a short point into the cup end of a large cup. Screw the long checkpoint into the flat end of the cup until the points touch. *Substitute the medium-length point for the long point if the interarch space is inadequate.* Prepare three sets of points.

2. Attach the three assembled checkpoint units to the completed bases, with the long checkpoint on the mandibular base. Position one in the anterior midline region and one on each side in the molar region. Use utility wax to temporarily

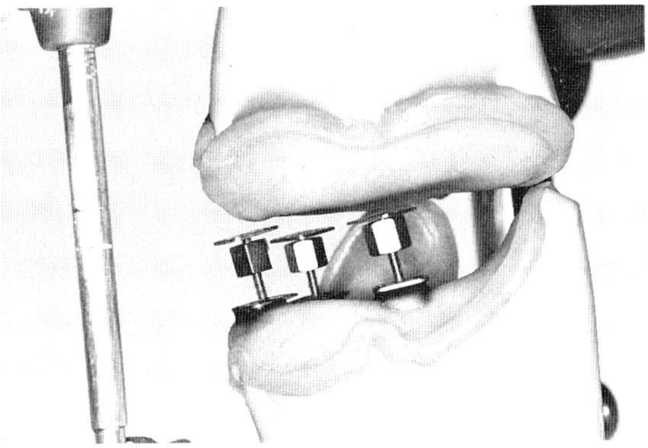

Fig. 8-19 A nub of utility wax is placed on the mandibular base to temporarily position the checkpoints.

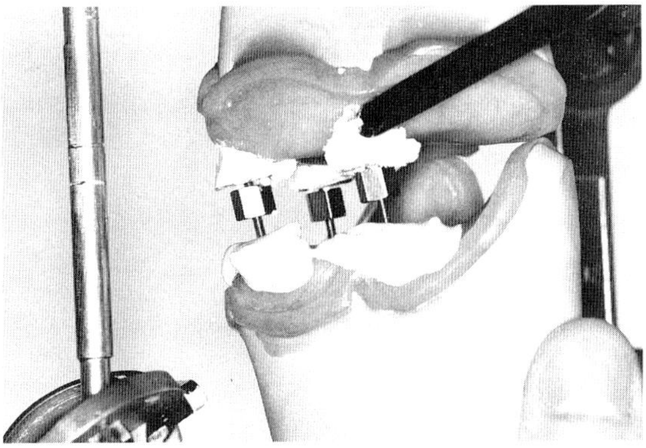

Fig. 8-20 Additional stone is painted on top of the grids for the maxillary points and the articulator is closed.

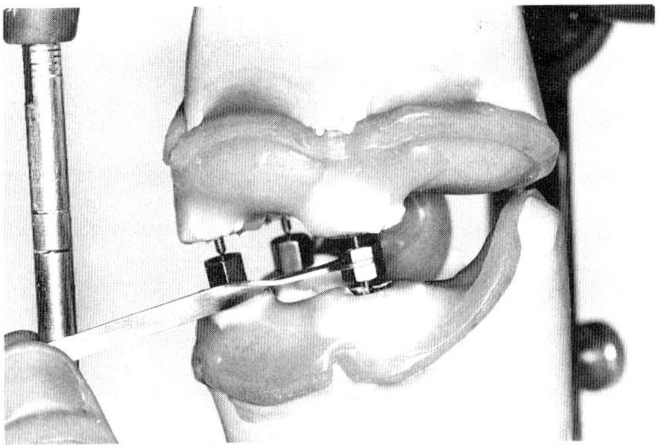

Fig. 8-21 Rotate the cup clockwise onto the long checkpoint.

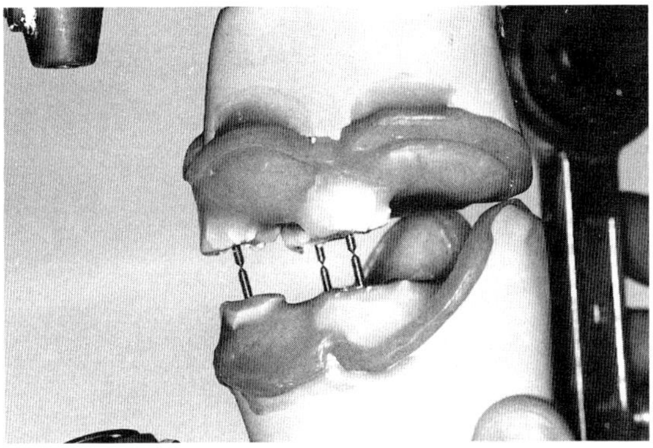

Fig. 8-22 The centric checkpoints must have precise contact on the articulator before they are checked in the mouth.

position the checkpoints (Fig. 8-19). Slant the checkpoints slightly forward so that they are approximately in line with the arc of closure of the mandible.

3. Attach the gridded, perforated bases of the long points to the mandibular base with stone and slurry. After the stone has set, seal the stone to the base with baseplate wax because the stone alone will not adhere to the acrylic resin.

4. Place additional stone on top of the grids of the maxillary points, and close the articulator (Fig. 8-20). After the stone has set, seal the stone to the maxillary base with baseplate wax.

5. Use the wrench to rotate the cup clockwise onto the long point (Fig. 8-21). This will free the maxillary point from contact with the mandibular point and allow the articulator to be opened. At this time, the cup can be rotated off the longer point. Close the articulator to verify that the checkpoints contact each other precisely (Fig. 8-22).

6. Remove the completed bases from the articulator, and place them in the mouth. Guide the patient into the centric jaw relation position. The checkpoints should come together the same as on the articulator (Fig. 8-23). All checkpoints must contact each other at the same instant in all three dimensions: anterior-posterior, superior-inferior, and mediolateral. If an error is seen in any dimension, a new centric jaw relation record should be made (Figs. 8-24a to c).

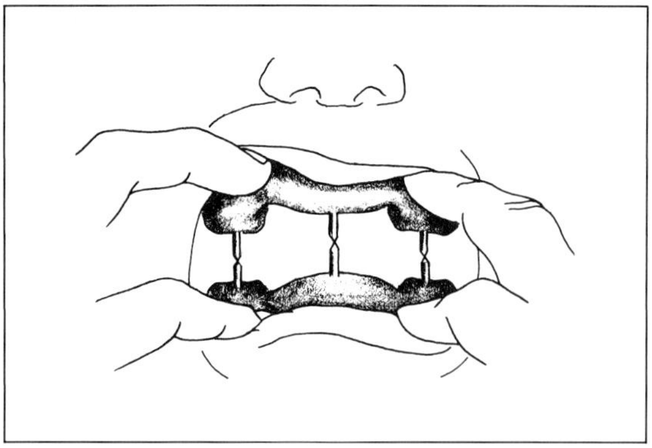

Fig. 8-23 The centric checkpoints come together in all three dimensions at the same instant.

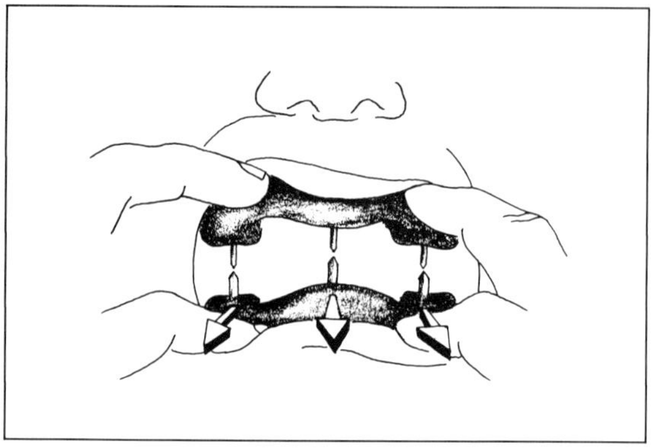

Fig. 8-24a Centric jaw relation is a three-dimensional relationship between the mandible and the maxilla. Each dimension is seen at the occlusal level when the checkpoints are used. An anterior-posterior error.

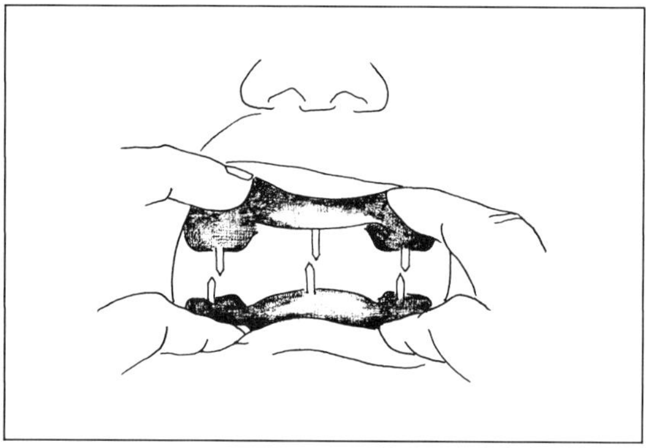

Fig. 8-24b A mediolateral error.

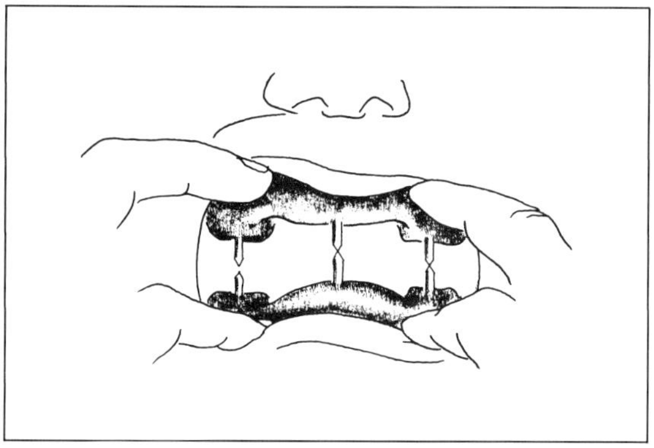

Fig. 8-24c A superior-inferior error.

Using checkpoints to reaccomplish centric jaw relation

1. Reposition the large cups on the long points with cup side up, and screw down until the tips of the points are flush with the tops of the cups.

2. Fill the cup concavity with baseplate wax. If one of the checkpoints touches before another in the superior-inferior dimension, the cup can be raised higher so that the opposing points will contact the wax at the same vertical level.

3. Return the checkpoints to the mouth and remake the centric jaw relation record. The checkpoints should make small indentations in the wax. Deep penetrations in the wax could significantly alter the vertical dimension of occlusion and make it difficult to verify the wax record (Figs. 8-25a and b). Repeat the centric closure to be sure that each checkpoint contacts the wax indentations at the same instant. If the initial record was in such gross error that the checkpoints do not touch the wax cups, additional wax should be added around the surfaces of the cup.

4. Remove the bases from the mouth and manually position the points in the opposing wax indentations. Secure the opposing bases using stone

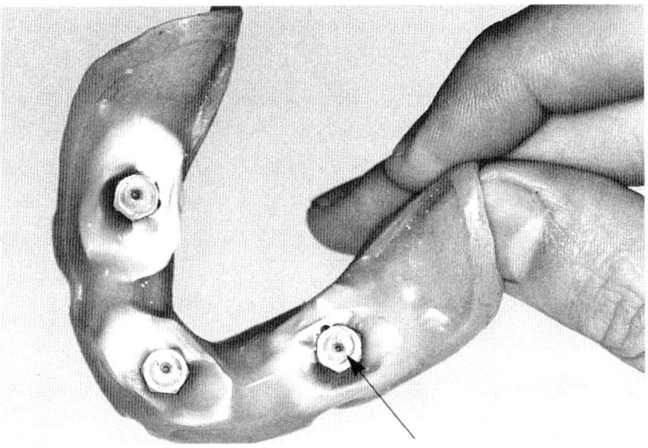

Fig. 8-25a A new centric jaw relation record is made with the checkpoints on the maxilla, making a record in the opposing wax cups. Indentations *(arrow)* in the wax cups made by opposing checkpoints.

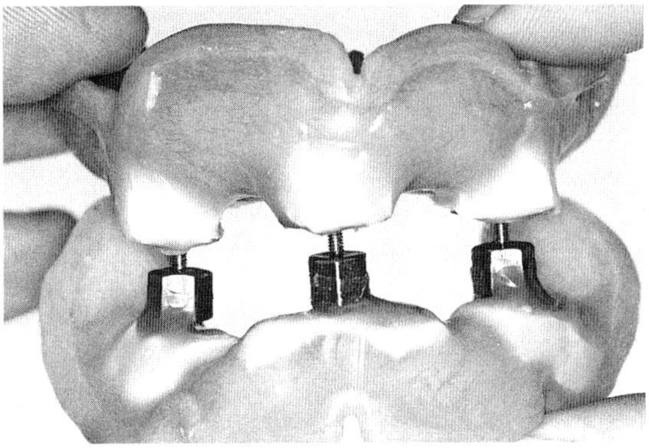

Fig. 8-25b Record bases are mounted via checkpoint indentations into the wax cups.

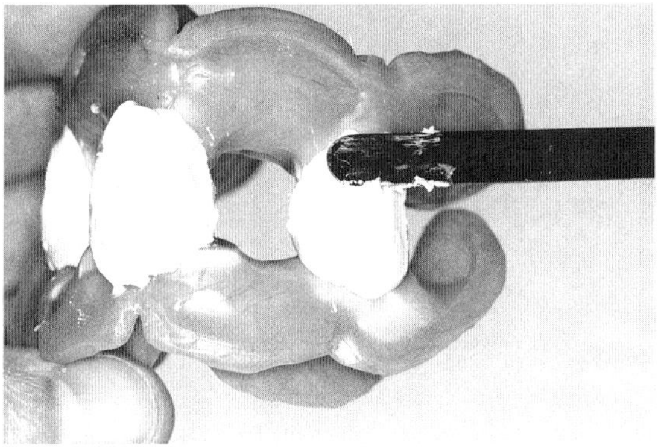

Fig. 8-26 Place a stone and slurry mixture between the points and wax cups to secure the bases.

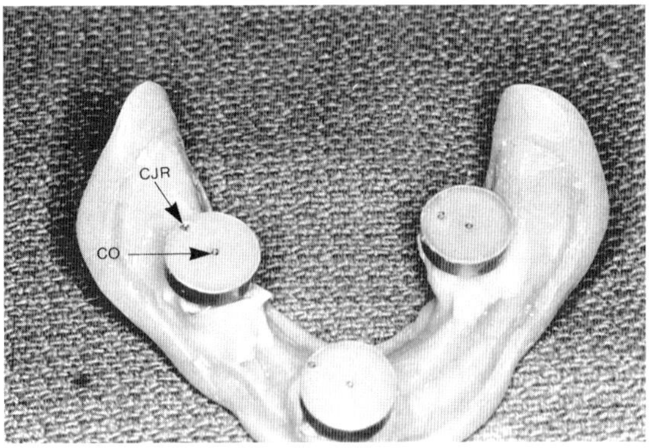

Fig. 8-27 The discrepancy between centric jaw relation *(CJR)* and centric occlusion *(CO)* is evident by their respective checkpoint contacts as shown in large wax cups.

and slurry (Fig. 8-26). Do not use sticky wax to secure the bases because it will melt the wax that is within the cup. Remove the mandibular mounting cast from the articulator and remount it using this new record.

5. Remove the wax cups from the mandibular baseplate and close the articulator. If this record was correct, the same error seen in the mouth should now be seen on the articulator.

6. Remove the short points from the maxillary base, clean them, and reattach them to the mandibular long checkpoints as previously described. Secure the short points to the maxillary base with stone and slurry as previously described. Rotate the cup onto the mandibular point and open the articulator. The checkpoints should again coincide. Return the points to the mouth to verify the centric jaw relation record. Repeat the verification procedures described until *no error* is evident.

The centric jaw relation record and articulator mounting have now been verified. The denture teeth can be set with the confidence that the casts are mounted correctly.

Visualization of the centric jaw relation–centric occlusion discrepancy

1. Have the patient sit upright in the dental chair without his head supported by the headrest while the checkpoints are still in the mouth.
2. Instruct the patient to close his teeth together *without any operator guidance,* and visualize how the mandibular points relate to the maxillary points (Fig. 8-27).

The discrepancy between the patient's centric jaw relation position and centric occlusion position is evident. This information is helpful in determining which type of posterior tooth form to use in the denture—anatomic or nonanatomic—and which position to use for setting the teeth to obtain maximum intercuspation.

Graser reported that one patient in his study had a 5-mm anterior-posterior discrepancy between centric jaw relation and centric occlusion.[19] Halperin and King reported that one of their patients had an approximately 3-mm anterior-posterior discrepancy between centric jaw relation and centric occlusion.[22] A decision must be made whether to use the centric jaw relation position or the centric occlusion position as the position of maximum intercuspation, or to use the centric jaw relation position as the starting position for the occlusal scheme, giving the patient the freedom to move anteriorly and/or laterally into a centric occlusion position. This is what some refer to as a "long and wide centric."

A thorough discussion of the selection and setting of posterior denture teeth is included in chapter 10.

References

1. Bonwill, W.G.A. The scientific articulation of the human teeth as founded on geometrical, mathematical and mechanical laws. Dent. Items of Interest, October 1899:617–643.
2. Monson, G.S. Applied mechanics to the theory of mandibular movements. Dent. Cosmos 74:1053, 1932.
3. Hanau, R.L. Articulation defined, analyzed and formulated. J. Am. Dent. Assoc. 13:1694, 1926.
4. Gysi, A. An analysis of the development of the articulator. J. Am. Dent. Assoc. 17:1401, 1930.
5. Atwood, D.A. A cephalometric study of the clinical rest position of the mandible. Part II. The variability of the rate of bone loss following the removal of occlusal contacts. J. Prosthet. Dent. 7:544, 1957.
6. Academy of Denture Prosthetics. Glossary of Prosthodontic Terms. 4th ed. St. Louis: C.V. Mosby Co., 1977.
7. Thompson, J.R. The rest position of the mandible and its significance to dental science. J. Am. Dent. Assoc. 33:151, 1946.
8. Tallgren, A. Changes in adult face height due to aging, wear and loss of teeth and prosthetic treatment. Acta Odontol. Scand. 15:1–112, 1957.
9. McGrane, H.F. Five basic principles of the McGrane full denture procedure. J. Florida Dent. Soc. 20:5–8, 1949.
10. Graser, G.N., Plekavich, E.J., and Espeland, M.A. Anthropometric measurements for anterior tooth position and vertical dimension of occlusion. Abstr. No. 719. J. Dent. Res. 65 (Special Issue March):249, 1986.
11. Posselt, V. Studies in the mobility of the human mandible. Acta Odontol. Scand. 10(Suppl. 10):1–160, 1952.
12. Temple, F.J. Een onderzoek naar de positie van de mandibula in centrale occlusia. Thesis. Gröningen, 1959.
13. Kydd, W.L., and Sander, A. A study of posterior mandibular movements from intercuspal occlusal position. J. Dent. Res. 40:419–425, 1961.
14. Beyron, H. Occlusal relations and mastication in Australian aborigines. Acta Odontol. Scand. 22:597, 1964.
15. Ingervall, B. Retruded contact position of the mandible. A comparison between children and adults. Odontol. Rev. 15:130–149, 1964.
16. Hodge, L.C., and Mahan, P.E. A study of mandibular movement from centric occlusion to maximum intercuspation. J. Prosthet. Dent. 18:19–30, 1967.
17. Helkimo, M., Ingervall, B., and Carlsson, G.E. Variation of retruded and muscular position of the mandible under different recording conditions. Acta Odontol. Scand. 29:423–437, 1971.
18. Agerberg, G. Avstand mellan olika ocklusionslagen och deras reproducer barket vid bettregistrering. Sven. Tandlak. Tidskr. 64:185–195, 1971.
19. Graser, G.N. Terminal hinge position or neuromuscular position: an evaluation of the edentulous. Part I. Maxillomandibular recordings. J. Prosthet. Dent. 36:491, 1976.
20. Graser, G.N. Terminal hinge position or neuromuscular position: an evaluation of the edentulous. Part II. Duplicate mandibular dentures. J. Prosthet. Dent. 37:1248, 1978.
21. Brewer, A.A. Prosthodontic research in progress at the School of Aerospace Medicine. J. Prosthet. Dent. 13:49, 1963.
22. Halperin, A.R., and King, R. Fabrication of a maxillary complete denture utilizing the neuromuscular position or centric occlusion. J. Am. Dent. Assoc. 100:67, 1980.

I don't care what method you use to transfer a centric jaw relation record to the articulator; the important thing is to know that the record is mounted on the articulator correctly before you proceed. To go ahead and place denture teeth upon the record bases before we know that the centric jaw relation is mounted correctly is a horrible waste of time. Yet this approach is taught in most dental schools: final impressions are made, temporary record bases are used to make a centric jaw relation record, teeth are then arranged, and then another centric jaw relation record is made. You continue to remake records until everybody gets tired of it. The dentures are then completed and another record and mounting is made on the day of insertion. The patient wears these dentures for awhile and then another centric record is made. I reason that it would be much better if I knew if the centric jaw relation record was right before I proceeded to set teeth; then I can eliminate all of these additional records and remounts. Successful use of any technique requires accurate and conscientious observation. The smallest errors may be seen and should be corrected.

Allen Brewer
(Personal communication)

Chapter 9

Anterior Tooth Selection and Arrangement

Anterior tooth selection and arrangement is an area of prosthodontics where art dominates science, where esthetics is the major concern, and where knowledge must be applied to create a pleasing appearance while simultaneously maintaining oral function. One important factor to consider is that while the teeth being selected and arranged are artificial, the resulting appearance must be natural.

Art is defined as "the conscious use of skill and creative imagination, especially in the production of esthetic objects."[1] The word *natural* is defined as "free from all artificiality and constraint and having an easy spontaneity that suggests nature rather than art."[1] When creating a complete denture, the art must disguise itself, leaving the patient with the appearance of having natural teeth.

It is important to remember who is being treated when it comes to the esthetics of complete dentures. The YMATO factors, as discussed in chapter 1, stand for *Y*ou, the patient, *M*e, the dentist, and *A*ll *T*hose *O*thers who will be concerned and affected by the selection and arrangement of the anterior teeth. The patient and dentist must work together to create dentures that are both pleasing and natural looking. The YMATO factor is applicable primarily to the patient and the dentist during this phase of denture fabrication. The dentist must learn to be an artist. This talent comes quickly to some; others take years to achieve it; some may never develop it. We all have varying degrees of artistic ability, and with practice and study it can be developed to a higher, more perceptive level. Dentists can develop their awareness of esthetics by spending more time observing natural teeth in photographs and in person. This will help them acquire a feeling for what is most pleasing and what is most unesthetic.

During treatment, patients must also be educated as to what will look natural and be most esthetic for them, especially if their previous denture has an unnatural appearance. The dentist can show a patient a scrapbook containing photographs and magazine clippings of other people—men and women, young and old—with dentures and with natural dentition.

Patients expect three basic things from their complete dentures: favorable appearance, comfort, and chewing ability. In a study where 7 sets of dentures were made for each of 12 patients by 7 dentists, each patient preferred the dentures that he thought looked the best.[2] Seven of the patients in this study selected the dentures that looked the best, even though they were not as comfortable as another set or not as easy to chew with.

In a second study, 64 patients were asked how their new complete dentures improved their self-image.[3] Nearly all the patients responded that the new dentures improved their appearance, increased self-confidence, and provided an overall sense of well-being.

The first and most important factor to be considered in anterior tooth selection and arrangement is *who the denture is being made for*. Only after this is understood can size of the teeth, mold (shape) of the teeth, shade of the teeth, and tooth material be considered. With proper attention to all of these factors, the natural, pleasing appearance that we are working towards can be achieved.

Patient evaluation: Who is the denture being made for?

One of the best ways to achieve patient satisfaction is to get the patient involved in the selection and arrangement of his teeth. One study has shown that when patients get involved in the decision-making process of tooth selection and arrangement, they enjoy increased satisfaction with their dentures.[4] Therefore, it is advantageous to encourage the patient's direct involvement and participation. How is this accomplished? If the patient is currently wearing dentures, ask him what he likes or dislikes about their appearance. What changes would the patient want? This questioning can begin at the first meeting (chapter 1) so that the patient can have adequate time to seriously consider things. If this is to be the first denture that the patient will have, there are likely some natural teeth present that have to be extracted. These few remaining teeth can be very helpful in the same way as existing dentures. Perhaps there are spaces between the patient's teeth, notches, grooves, or restorations that the patient would like recreated in the new denture. An impression of the natural teeth before their extraction can be helpful. Any old photographs of the patient that show the position of the anterior teeth are helpful. Our goal is to gather as much information as possible so that the dentures we make have a natural appearance and are accepted by the patient.

However, we do not want to show the patient the mold guide and have him select the teeth. Seeing that many variations would only confuse him. In fact, it is only after the teeth have been arranged on the denture base with a wax gingival matrix and the dentist approves of their appearance that the patient has his first opportunity to observe the teeth.

Anterior tooth selection

There are four main considerations when selecting anterior teeth: *(1)* tooth size, *(2)* tooth mold, *(3)* color, and *(4)* tooth material. Following are conventionally used guidelines for the selection of anterior denture teeth. The information given should be used simply as *guidelines*, not as *rules*. Use your creativity and imagination in selecting teeth.

Guidelines for selection of tooth size

The dimension, or size, of the individual anterior teeth as well as the combined width of the six anterior teeth are important. There are two dimensions to consider: *(1)* the mesiodistal width, and *(2)* the incisogingival length.

Mesiodistal width

An estimated total width of the six maxillary anterior teeth may be obtained by dividing 3.3 into the greatest bizygomatic width.[5] House and Loop's rule of dividing the bizygomatic width (measured in millimeters) by 16 provides a starting point for the width of the maxillary central incisor.[6] Measure the bizygomatic width with a face-bow, and divide this number by 16. The lateral incisors are approximately 2 mm narrower and the canine 1 mm narrower than the central incisors.[7] This formula should provide the overall width of the six maxillary anteriors.

Another method for selecting the anterior teeth is to mark the corners of the mouth on a wax rim. The measurement from one side to the other will represent the combined width of the six maxillary anterior teeth.

Incisogingival length

The wax rim is also used to mark the height of the smile line. Instruct the patient to smile, and place a line on the rim at the point to which the lip elevates. This will help determine the length of the tooth required. As a general guideline, the maxillary lip comes close to the gingival neck of the tooth when a patient smiles broadly (Fig. 9-1).

House and Loop also suggested using facial measurements to help select the length of the maxillary central incisors.[6] Measure the distance from the hairline to the gnathion in millimeters, and divide this number by 16. This will give you the suggested length of the maxillary central incisor. Obviously, not all patients show as much of their maxillary

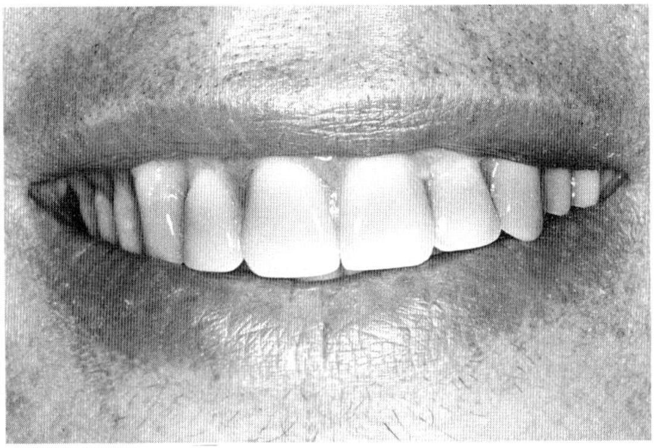

Fig. 9-1 As a general guideline, the maxillary lip rises to the gingival neck of the tooth when a patient smiles broadly.

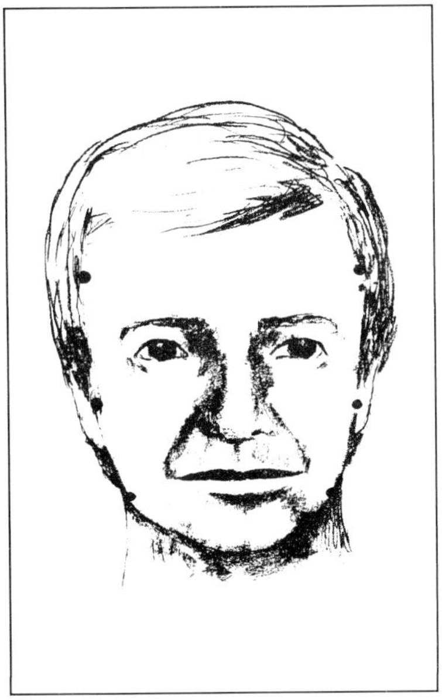

Fig. 9-2 *(right)* The face form is identified by connecting the following points on the patient's face: the forehead, the zygomatic arch, and the angle of the mandible.

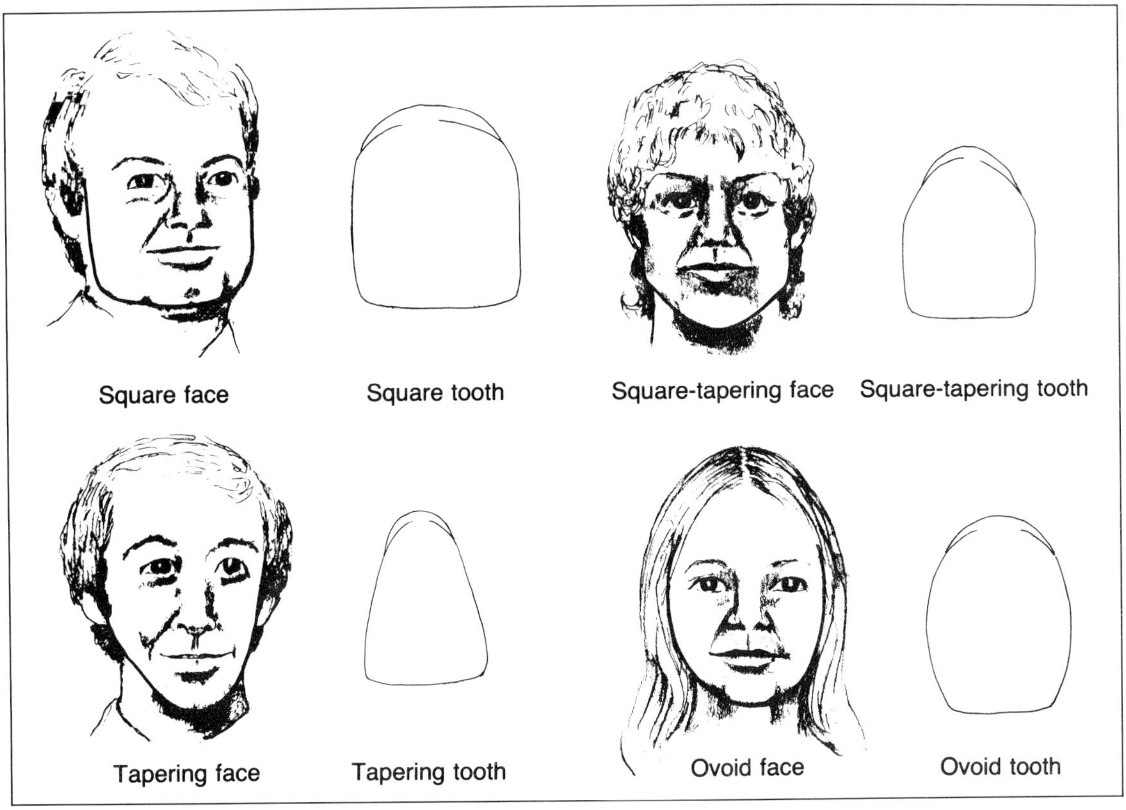

Fig. 9-3 The four basic types of face forms should be considered when selecting the maxillary central incisors.

teeth when they smile, but the occlusion rim can be a starting point for tooth selection.

The manufacturers of denture teeth usually relate the size of the mandibular anterior teeth to the maxillary anterior teeth. Therefore, once maxillary anterior teeth have been selected, the mold guide lists which mandibular anterior teeth are appropriate.

Guidelines for selection of tooth mold (shape)

Outline form of tooth

The outline form, or shape, of the anterior teeth was first considered important by Williams[8] and House and Loop.[6] They classified the outline forms, or shapes, of the face and selected anterior denture teeth which were in harmony with the facial form. Their face form is identified by connecting the following points on the lateral aspect of the face: the forehead, the zygomatic arch, and the angle of the mandible (Fig. 9-2).

There are four basic shapes that a person's face can have: *(1)* square, *(2)* square tapering, *(3)* tapering, and *(4)* ovoid (Fig. 9-3). The shape of the maxillary central incisor should resemble the shape of the face if it were placed upside down (inverted). For example, a person with a square-shaped face may look best with a square-shaped maxillary central incisor.

This method of tooth selection became known as the *geometric theory*. Most dental manufacturers base their entire systems of tooth selection on these typal face forms. However, the maxillary central incisors of patients with natural teeth are not necessarily the inverted facial form. Wright found that 60.7% of his subjects had natural maxillary central incisors that were not the inverted facial form.[9] Bell examined the maxillary central incisors of 31 subjects whose natural teeth were considered esthetically acceptable.[10] There was no correlation between the form of the face and the form of the maxillary central incisors. However, although an ovoid tooth may not always be found with an ovoid-shaped face, for example, from an artistic point of view such an approach may be reasonable. When all of the patient's natural teeth are missing, facial form can be a valuable guideline. Also, there are times when we can improve upon nature—orthodontists do this every day. Therefore, a tooth that complements facial form may provide a very natural, pleasing appearance.

Tooth curvature

A tooth may curve in both a mesiodistal and an incisogingival direction. The incisogingival curvature and mesiodistal curvature of the teeth selected can complement the profile curvatures of the face (Fig. 9-4). One tooth manufacturer* labels its tooth molds *F* (flat) or C (curved), according to their labial surfaces.

It is a good idea to select anterior teeth that are a little larger than you might need so that you can reshape them for cosmetic purposes. The concept employed here is that within the tooth selected is "another tooth," which can be reshaped to the desired form for that individual patient. A common mistake is to select anterior denture teeth that are too small. The stock denture tooth should be regarded as a place to start. The dentist should consider it his responsibility to recontour and reshape each tooth to provide a more individual and natural composition for each patient.

Guidelines for selection of tooth shade

The three dimensions of color to consider are *hue*, the attribute of colors that permits them to be classed as red, yellow, blue, and so on; *value*, the relative brightness or darkness of a color; and *chroma*, the amount or concentration of the color (hue). Hue, value, and chroma are terms that relate to color in general, and are also very important when we discuss tooth selection. Hue is basically the color of an object.

In most shade guides today, yellow is the predominant hue. The other colors play a much smaller role. The value increases as an object be-

*Lactona Corp., Hatfield, Pa.

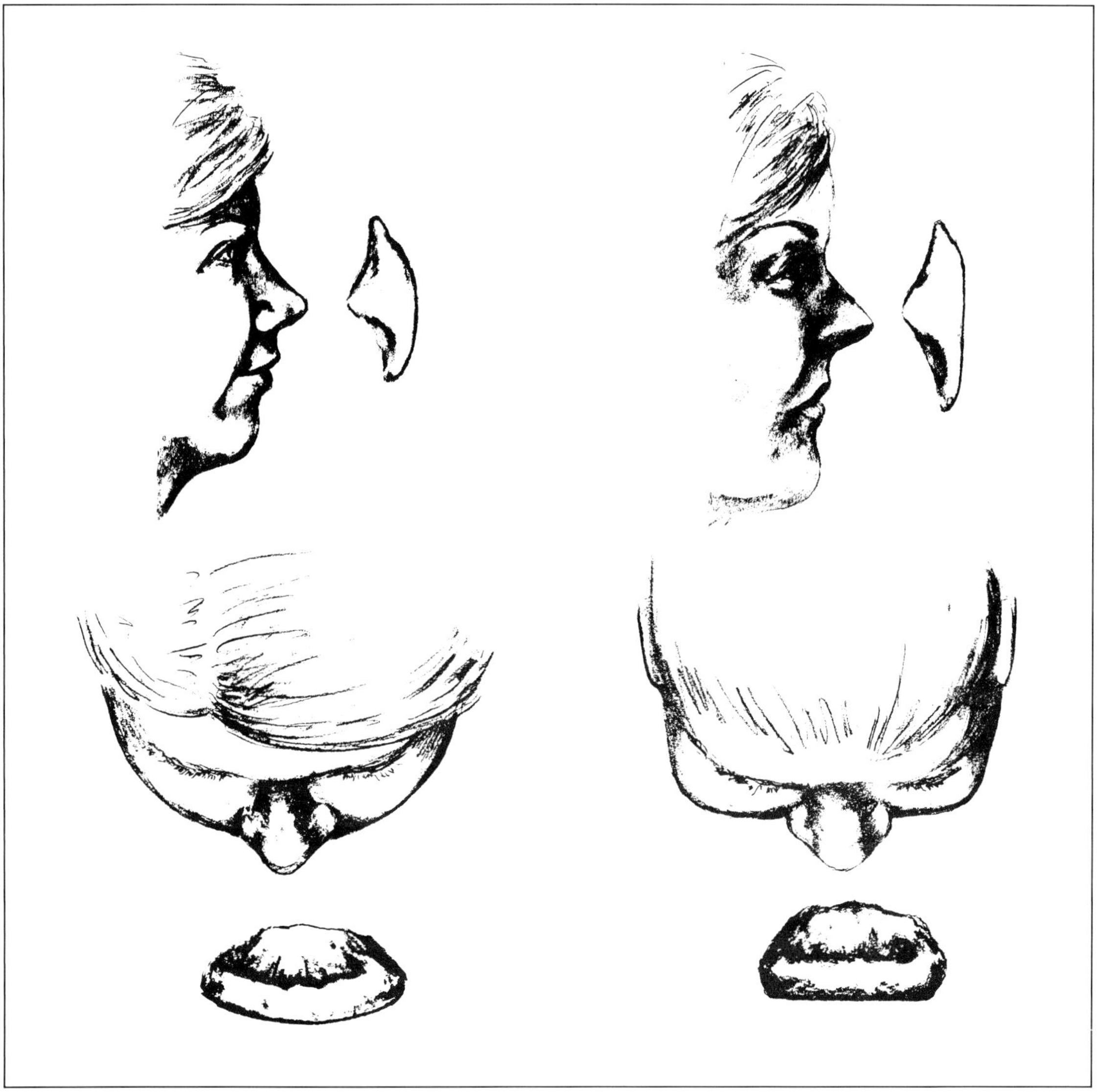

Fig. 9-4 The incisogingival and mesiodistal curvatures of the tooth selected can complement the profile curvature of the face.

comes lighter or more nearly white. As people advance in age, their teeth tend to become darker, or decrease in value. Chroma (saturation) is the amount of hue in a color. Because yellow is the predominant hue, chroma refers to the amount of yellow in each tooth.

In the fabrication of complete dentures it is important to use teeth that possess different shades rather than merely one shade. Shades can also vary within the same tooth, which helps to create a more natural, pleasing appearance.

When selecting a shade for complete dentures,

do not ask the patient to look at a shade guide and select what he would like. Instead, select a shade based on some of the upcoming guidelines, remembering that about 8% of the male population is color blind so a female assistant may be helpful in selecting a shade, especially for removable partial dentures. There is no scientific formula for selection of tooth color for the edentulous patient, but these guidelines may be used:

1. Each manufacturer offers different shades, and it is wise to use several shade guides when choosing a shade.
2. With advancing age, teeth become less brilliant or of lower value. They become yellower and grayer.
3. As a rule, the darker the complexion of the individual, the lower the value of tooth to select.
4. The most important factor to examine is the complexion of the patient versus his hair or eye color, because of relative proximity and amount of skin. Hold the shade tabs to the patient's skin near his lips. A test that may be helpful involves slowly closing your eyes. The shade that disappears first is the closest to the complexion of the patient.[11]
5. Breaking up the color of the anterior teeth can be accomplished by selecting teeth of different shades. This can create the illusion of greater depth and naturalness. Using a lateral incisor that is a shade lighter than the central incisor and canine can provide a more natural appearance. The canines are usually darker than the central incisors.
6. Generally, when selecting the mandibular anterior tooth shade, the same shade selected for the maxillary anterior teeth may be used. For a Class III (prognathic) patient, less brilliant (lower value) mandibular anterior teeth would not appear to stand out as much as lighter shade teeth. Conversely, lighter shade teeth would be used for a Class II (retrognathic) patient to create the illusion that the teeth are more anterior than they really are.

Guidelines for selection of tooth material

The following materials are available for selection of anterior denture teeth: *(1)* conventional acrylic resin, *(2)* interpenetrating polymer network (IPN) acrylic resin, *(3)* composite resin, and *(4)* porcelain. Deciding which type of teeth to use is based upon esthetics; wear resistance and hardness; noise made when teeth contact; ease of setting, repairing, and processing; and bond of teeth to acrylic resin denture base material. Each material's advantages and disadvantages must be weighed carefully, based upon personal preference and objectives. A brief discussion of each material will highlight some of the advantages, disadvantages, indications, and contraindications for their use.

Conventional acrylic resin teeth

The newer acrylic resin teeth are far superior to the originals because of improvements in the chemical nature and processing of the teeth. The first acrylic resin teeth that were made got a "bad name" because they wore and discolored quickly. The newer resins are cross-linked, more dense, and much more wear resistant than the first acrylic resin teeth. Acrylic resin teeth can be ground very thin to fit into tight spaces without compromising the strength of their bond to the acrylic resin denture base material. The occlusal and facial surfaces of the teeth are easily polished. The teeth are also easily reshaped for esthetic purposes. In function, acrylic resin teeth do not make much noise when they come together. Acrylic resin teeth can wear with time, however, and are also subject to abrasion with inappropriate scrubbing or cleaning (see chapter 13).

*Interpenetrating polymer network (IPN) acrylic resin teeth**

This tooth material is a nonfilled, highly cross-linked copolymer with an interpenetrating polymer network.[12] The relationships between four component materials have been optimized by computer studies, and these materials have been combined by sophisticated production processes into an interpenetrating polymer network. The material is

*Dentsply International, Inc., York, Pa.

formed when the first polymer is cross-linked into a three-dimensional network prior to formation of the second polymer, and when that second polymer is formed in such a fashion that it, too, is a cross-linked, three-dimensional network. IPN teeth can be ground, and because they are made of acrylic resin, they bond well to the denture bases. Because of its polymer structure, the IPN material is harder, more abrasion resistant, more stain resistant, and more heat resistant than conventional resins. There are no disadvantages to substituting IPN teeth for conventional cross-linked acrylic resin teeth. IPN teeth are set up and used exactly as are conventional acrylic resin teeth.

Composite resin teeth

Vivosit* teeth (or Orthosit* posterior teeth) consist of an organic filler and a liquid matrix based on a modified Bowen resin.[13] Both the liquid matrix and the organic filler contain approximately 20% pyrolytic silicium dioxide, which is used as a thickening and strengthening agent. Pyrolytic silicium dioxide is a material that has a particle size in the range of 10 to 400 Å, which is less than the wavelength of visible light. This very small particle size leads to a cosmetically acceptable material. Porcelain denture teeth have the disadvantage that pins must be used for mechanical retention to the acrylic resin denture base material. The acrylic resin teeth, as mentioned, bond chemically to the acrylic resin denture base, but they have the disadvantage of greater wear potential than porcelain teeth. The Vivosit tooth has significantly greater wear resistance than conventional acrylic resin and will still chemically bond to the acrylic resin denture base materials. Again, as with the IPN material, Vivosit teeth can be used as a substitute for the conventional acrylic resin teeth.

Porcelain teeth

Porcelain denture teeth have the highest wear resistance of any of the denture tooth materials. They are also the most stain resistant. The disadvantages are that for patients who have neuromuscular coordination problems or nervous habits of clicking their teeth together, porcelain teeth will make much more noise upon contact than acrylic resin teeth. When interarch space is a problem, porcelain anterior teeth have retentive pins in the area where the teeth would have to be ground in. Porcelain teeth are also subject to chipping or fracture.

*Ivoclar (USA) Inc., San Marcos, Calif.

Making the final tooth selection

Manufacturers distribute mold and shade guides to help in the tooth selection process. The criteria and guidelines given assist in the selection of teeth. Keeping all this information in mind, the dentist should approach the patient using creativity and imagination. Most importantly, look at the denture teeth available and select some that will look good in the patient's mouth. The final decision as to their acceptability will not come until the try-in. Do not merely depend upon the guidelines for tooth selection that have been discussed.

Although we do want the patient's input regarding anterior tooth selection, do not encourage the patient to select the teeth with you. A patient would be looking at the manufacturer's shade and mold guides with an untrained eye, unable to project the appearance of the teeth in his own mouth. When a shade guide is held up in front of a patient, he is apt to select a shade that will be too light—too white. It is difficult enough for a dentist to select a shade or mold without confusing the issue through patient involvement. When the teeth are eventually set up and properly arranged on the record bases, the patient can see them within their future environment—within the framework of face and mouth. At this time, the appropriate gingival contour should be waxed around the necks of the teeth to help create a natural look.

Anterior tooth arrangement

Once the anterior teeth have been selected, the challenge is to position them on the denture base so as to defy their detection as being artificial. Arranging the anterior teeth while the patient is present can be worthwhile for both the patient and dentist. The patient has a sense of personal involvement and sees that the dentures are being personalized for him and actually made by the dentist, while the dentist has the opportunity to check the anterior tooth positions before the posterior teeth are set. If time does not permit, however, the anterior teeth can be arranged by the dentist or laboratory technician prior to the anterior tooth try-in. Because the maxillary occlusion rim was removed from the record base to set the centric relation checkpoints, it is imperative that the dentist arrange at least the two maxillary and mandibular central incisors while the patient is present. This will give the dentist or laboratory technician ample information to complete the anterior tooth setup for a try-in. The midline of the upper face should also be marked upon the maxillary record base and then transferred to the maxillary mounting cast by scribing a mark upon it.

Horizontal and vertical overlap of the anterior teeth

The amount of horizontal and vertical overlap of the anterior teeth is determined by esthetics, phonetics, and function. The anterior teeth are positioned so that an appropriate amount of both the maxillary and mandibular teeth show. At the vertical dimension of occlusion selected, a certain amount of maxillary and mandibular teeth will show during rest or function (speech, smiling, and so on). The proportionality of maxillary or mandibular tooth to be displayed in the completed denture is first considered when the tentative vertical dimension of occlusion is established. The final evaluation of the proportionality of tooth display occurs during the try-in visits. After the teeth have been set for esthetic purposes, their position is then tested phonetically (see chapter 11). The degree of vertical and horizontal overlap affects the amount of incisal guidance. The smaller the horizontal overlap and the greater the vertical overlap, the steeper the posterior cusp height should be if a balanced occlusion is desired (see chapter 10). Increasing the vertical overlap of the anterior teeth will increase the display of anterior teeth.

Esthetic arrangement of the anterior teeth

The arrangement of the anterior teeth should be individualized to the patient's cosmetic needs. The bottom line is that the teeth must look like they belong in the patient's mouth. The time devoted to arranging the anterior teeth is often greater than for any of the other steps in denture fabrication. This is primarily because this procedure is not simply a technique but also an art.

Frush and Fisher suggested guidelines for selection and arrangement of anterior teeth based upon the patient's age, sex, and personality.[14–16] Although these guidelines are not absolute, they do offer helpful suggestions for enhancing the cosmetic appearance of many patients' teeth. Techniques for harmonizing the patient's teeth with age, sex, or personality are discussed below. Contributing techniques are also listed for clarity.

Age

Age is often revealed by the amount of maxillary and/or mandibular teeth that shows during rest or function. With increasing age, the amount of maxillary central incisors exposed when the lips are gently parted decreases from 3+ mm at age 29 to no tooth showing at 60 years of age.[17] The opposite occurs for the mandibular incisors, with approximately 0.5 mm showing at age 29 and 3 mm showing at age 60.

Some patients presenting for complete denture treatment have badly worn existing natural teeth or dentures. Often their vertical dimension of occlusion has "collapsed," and they are overclosed. During rest, speech, or smiling, these patients may show little or no tooth. In making new dentures for this type of patient, the amount of tooth that will be displayed will partly be a function of the vertical dimension of occlusion selected for the dentures. If the vertical dimension of occlusion is increased, more of the teeth will show. Before accepting this as appropriate, the patient must be advised of the esthetic change. His approval, and the approval of family members and friends, must be considered. It may be quite inappropriate to have an elderly patient show the amount of tooth

Table 9-1 Tooth characteristics by sex

Masculine characteristics	Feminine characteristics
Flat labial surface—mesiodistally and incisogingivally	Curved labial surface—mesiodistally and incisogingivally
Broad arch form; central incisors slightly turned in on the mesial side	Tapered or curved arch form; central incisors turned in at the distoincisal edge
Canines more prominent and turned out at the incisal edge	Canines arranged to appear turned in at the incisal edge (inclined palatally)
Sharper mesioincisal and distoincisal angles	Rounded mesioincisal and distoincisal angles
Incisal edge of lateral incisor often at same level as central incisor	Incisal edge of lateral incisor raised compared to central incisor and canine
Broad lateral incisors	Narrow lateral incisors

that a 30-year-old would display. On the other hand, some chronologically older patients do not appear to be their age, and their teeth can help provide a more youthful appearance.

Frush and Fisher state that the dignity of advancing age can be successfully portrayed in the denture by careful tooth color selection and mold refinement.[16] By varying the long axis of the teeth, using diastemata, and grinding the incisal edges, the appearance of the anterior teeth can be transformed from youthful to advanced in age. A compromise between the two can be developed for middle age. Equally important is the matrix around the teeth. In youth, the interdental papillae are pointed, closely adapted to the tooth, and stippled. With age, they become shortened, blunted, edematous, and smooth, with signs of gingival recession around the necks of some of the teeth. Natural teeth wear with age in most patients, and this wear can be simulated by grinding the incisal edges of the denture teeth. Chips or notches can also be placed on the incisal edges. The interproximal surfaces near the gingival margin can be ground to provide a tooth with more depth, again simulating the effects of age.

The wax matrix around the teeth can be changed to reveal more or less of the teeth and to alter the shape of the teeth to square, square tapering, tapering, or ovoid. It can also be changed to match the age of the patient.

The labial surfaces of the anterior teeth can be roughened to remove surface gloss. This can lower the value of the denture tooth and improve the esthetics.

Sex

For an anterior tooth arrangement to appear feminine, the individual teeth must have feminine characteristics. These teeth will have softer anatomic features. They will have a spherical form, which often can be created only by individually reshaping the interproximal and incisal surfaces. The incisal edges must follow a curve, which suggests softness. The position of the anterior teeth can also suggest femininity. An anterior mesial rotation of the lateral incisor, combined with a slightly cervical inclination of one of the central incisors and a canine with its cervical portion facing outward compared to the incisal edge, provides a feminine arrangement.

A more masculine appearance is achieved by a more square or cuboidal tooth form. The incisal edges are flat, with less of a curve to the edges of the six anterior teeth. The central incisors can be arranged so that the incisal edges are in line with each other, or even and level at the mesial edges to create an even more masculine arrangement. The lateral incisors are rotated in at the mesial edges, and the canines are more vertical, cervical

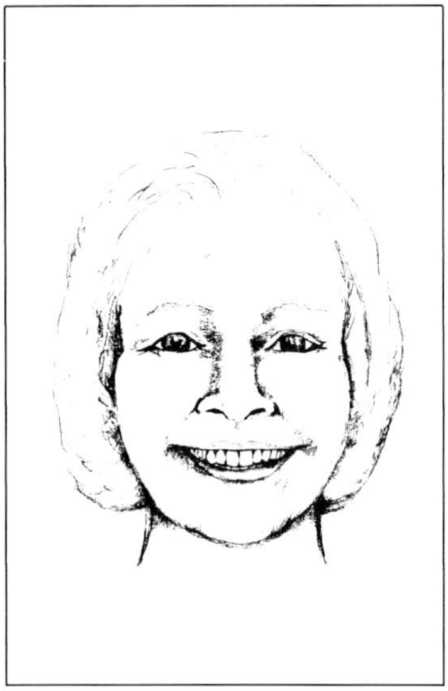

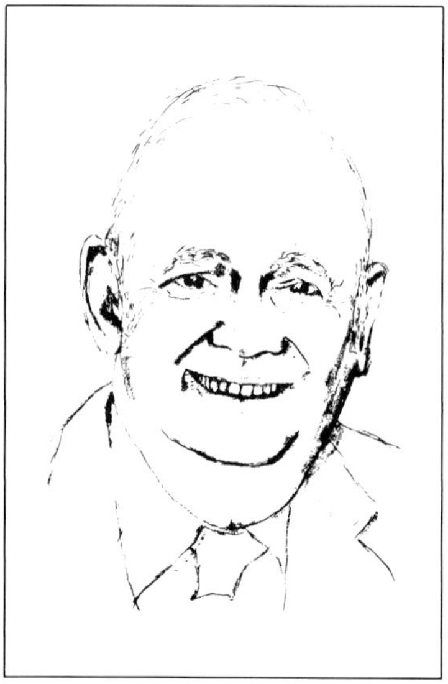

Fig. 9-5a *(left)* A delicate arrangement of teeth.

Fig. 9-5b *(right)* A more vigorous arrangement of teeth.

incisally. See Table 9-1 for an outline of masculine and feminine tooth characteristics.

Personality

Attempting to position and shape the teeth to complement the patient's personality involves getting to know the patient. Our goal is to express the individuality of that particular patient. Frush and Fisher have used a "personality spectrum" ranging from delicate to medium pleasing to vigorous.[16] The delicate personality is fragile and frail, while the vigorous is hard and aggressive. These personalities have ranges and blend with the medium personality, which is more moderate and somewhat robust. A small segment of the population has a delicate personality, while a slightly larger group is vigorous. The vast majority is in the medium range but tends toward the delicate or vigorous. The difference between the delicate and vigorous arrangements can be seen in Fig. 9-5a and b.

Each tooth is important in portraying personality. Again, the wax matrix is extremely important in the expression of personality because it controls the cervical one half to one third of the tooth contour. The central incisors play the dominant role in establishing the personality, followed by the canines and finally the lateral incisors. Although we are speaking about anterior tooth selection, the premolars also play an important role in the development of a natural appearance. A variation in their shade as well as in the long axes of their alignment contributes to the overall success of the final dentures.

Protrusive record

During the initial try-in of the anterior teeth, a protrusive record is made. Once the horizontal condylar inclinations are known, this information will be of value in the selection of the posterior teeth, which is described in the next chapter. The protrusive record is made at the early stage so that the posterior teeth can be set more precisely and in better harmony with the movements that will occur in the mouth. Follow these steps:

1. Insert the maxillary and mandibular record bases into the mouth. Rehearse with the patient to protrude his mandible approximately 3 to 4 mm anterior to the centric jaw relation position. It is often necessary to give the patient a hand mirror to help visualize the necessary movement.
2. Soften a sheet of baseplate wax and double

its thickness. Adapt the double-thick baseplate wax to the mandibular posterior tooth area bilaterally. (Block posterior monoplane teeth can be set at this time for convenience in making a stable record.) At least two sheets of wax are necessary for this record because of the Christensen phenomenon: the posterior teeth separate because the condyles move downward, creating a space between the posterior teeth.[18]

3. Gently heat the wax with an alcohol torch or wax instrument, and insert it in the mouth. Stabilize the mandibular base with your forefingers and instruct and guide the patient into the rehearsed position. Remove the record and chill both bases in cold water.

4. Secure the mandibular base to the mounting cast, and secure the wax rims together using sticky wax. Do not secure the maxillary base to the mounting cast.

5. Loosen the condylar lock and centric mechanisms on the articulator, and fit the mounting cast into the maxillary base as well as you can. Rotate the condylar mechanism to different degrees until the mounting cast fits into the maxillary base as precisely as possible.

6. For future reference, write directly on the maxillary mounting the condylar inclination values that were achieved.

Summary

The time devoted to selecting and arranging anterior teeth for the edentulous patient is usually much greater than for any other procedure, such as making impressions or determining maxillomandibular jaw relations. This is primarily because the predominant factor involved in selecting and setting anterior teeth is art, not science. We are trying to create a natural appearance using something artificial. We want to please not only the patient and ourselves, but all those others with whom the patient may come in contact.

We must get the patient involved to find out his likes and dislikes. We must use all the clues available to us as to what his natural teeth were like. We may not always want to make everything look as it did, for perhaps we can improve upon the natural dentition, but it does provide a very good place to start.

After various guides have been used to select the proper size, shape, and color, some average values can be very beneficial to the initial arrangement of the teeth when no other guidance is available. This first tooth arrangement has to be modified and individualized for that particular patient, but it does provide some preliminary scientific basis in what is otherwise an extremely challenging phase of denture fabrication for even the most artistic dentist.

A protrusive record is made at this stage so that the condylar inclination can be set on the instrument prior to arranging the posterior teeth.

References

1. Webster's New Collegiate Dictionary. Springfield, Mass.: G & C Merriam Co., 1977.
2. Brewer, A.A., Reibel, P.R., and Nassif, N.J. Comparison of zero degree and anatomic teeth on complete dentures. J. Prosthet. Dent. 17:28–35, 1967.
3. Straus, R., et al. Behavioral factors and denture status. J. Prosthet. Dent. 37:264–273, 1977.
4. Guckes, A.D., Smith, D.E., and Swoope, G.C. Counseling and related factors influencing satisfaction with dentures. J. Prosthet. Dent. 39:259, 1978.
5. Hickey, J.C., and Zarb, G.A. (eds.) Boucher's Prosthodontic Treatment for Edentulous Patients. St. Louis: C.V. Mosby Co., 1980.
6. House, M.M., and Loop, J.L. Form and color harmony in the dental art. Monograph: Whittier, Calif., 1939.
7. Krajicek, D.D. Personalized acrylic resin anterior teeth. J. Prosthet. Dent. 6:29–36, 1956.
8. Williams, J.L. The temperamental selection of artificial teeth, a fallacy. Dent. Digest 20:63, 1914.
9. Wright, W.H. Selection and arrangement of artificial teeth for complete prosthetic dentures. J. Am. Dent. Assoc. 23:2291, 1936.
10. Bell, R.A. The geometric theory of selection of artificial teeth: Is it valid? J. Prosthet. Dent. 97:637, 1978.
11. Wehner, P.J., Hickey, J.C., and Boucher, C.O. Selection of artificial teeth. J. Prosthet. Dent. 18:222–232, 1967.
12. Smith, R.A., Dentsply International, Inc., York, Pa. Personal communications, 1983.
13. Michl, R. Isosit, a new dental material. Quintessence Int. 9:1, 1978.
14. Frush, J.P., and Fisher, R.D. How dentogenic restorations interpret the sex factor. J. Prosthet. Dent. 6:160–172, 1956.
15. Frush, J.P., and Fisher, R.D. How dentogenics interpret the personality factor. J. Prosthet. Dent. 6:441–449, 1956.
16. Frush, J.P., and Fisher, R.D. The age factor in dentogenics. J. Prosthet. Dent. 7:5–13, 1957.
17. Vig, R.G., and Brundo, G.C. The kinetics of anterior tooth display. J. Prosthet. Dent. 39:502–504, 1978.
18. Christensen, C. The problem of the bite. Dent. Cosmos 47:1184–1195, 1905.

In making complete dentures for over 10,000 patients who were already wearing dentures, I found four faults in common. These are as follows: *(1)* inadequate coverage of residual ridges by the denture bases; *(2)* inadequate maxillomandibular records—whatever relationship the patient has was acquired by moving over to it, not up to it; *(3)* the wrong teeth in the wrong place—usually teeth that were too small set too far back and that were related only to an articulator and occlusion rims, not to the patient; and *(4)* inadequate assessment of the interocclusal distance.

If I were to assign the greatest importance to any one fact, I would say that the patient should look comfortable, and he cannot really look comfortable unless he *is* comfortable. So, we cannot underestimate the importance of adequate impressions, an accurate maxillomandibular record, and proper assessment of the vertical dimension of occlusion. If these steps are not adequately accomplished, good esthetics, comfort, and chewing ability will be missing.

I devote more time to esthetics in all of its manifestations than to any other phase of denture construction. I have produced the desired result in one-half hour, and I have taken as much as one week. I have completed the dentures and then altered the selection and arrangement of some or all of the teeth a day, a week, or months after the insertion.

Allen Brewer
(From: Selection of denture teeth for esthetics and function. J. Prosthet. Dent. 23:371, 1970.)

Chapter 10

Posterior Tooth Selection and Arrangement

As much as artistic ability plays a role in the selection and setting of anterior teeth, *technical ability* is the primary factor in the arrangement of posterior teeth. The selection of the posterior teeth is not based on hard-and-fast rules, but rather upon some criteria that will allow for patient function along with a balanced occlusion when necessary.

This chapter will describe what factors should be taken into consideration when selecting posterior denture teeth, be they anatomic or nonanatomic, procelain or acrylic resin. The rationale for arranging a balanced occlusion versus a nonbalanced occlusion will also be discussed. The technical procedures in arranging posterior anatomic and nonanatomic denture teeth will be reviewed. "Lingualized" (lingual cusp) occlusion will also be discussed.

Although the dentist may not set the posterior teeth, he is responsible for the manner in which they function when inserted in the patient's mouth. He should have a good understanding of the correct place of orientation, compensating curve, incisal guidance, and other components that may affect the occlusion of the dentures.

Anatomic versus nonanatomic teeth

Balance versus nonbalance

The question of whether dentures should have a balanced occlusion or not has been debated for many years. Today, there are still no objective studies that strongly support either the balanced or nonbalanced occlusion. Brewer found that when fabricating complete dentures with anatomic teeth (33°) and a balanced occlusion as compared with nonanatomic teeth (0°) set on an articulator used as a hinge, patients had no preference, and in fact did not realize that they had two different types of dentures.[1]

In a longitudinal study comparing dentures made with a "complex technique" and those made with a standard technique, Hickey, Ellinger, and coworkers found no significant differences over five years in denture retention and stability, condition of closure, and bone loss.[2–6] The complex technique involved a hinge axis location for face-bow transfer to a semiadjustable articulator. Eccentric records were made and the teeth were adjusted to a fully balanced occlusion. The standard technique involved no face-bow transfer, and the teeth were arranged and corrected in centric occlusion only. No attempt was made to balance the occlusion. One must keep in mind that the dentists fabricating the dentures were very experienced in treating edentulous patients and did adjust the occlusion intraorally at the time of insertion for the standard technique.

It would appear that balanced occlusion is not a factor for normal function, such as mastication. However, because stability and retention can be affected by parafunctional movements such as bruxism or lateral contacts, it might be beneficial to have simultaneous contact of both sides of the occlusion upon closure in various positions, especially if the individual is a difficult denture patient.

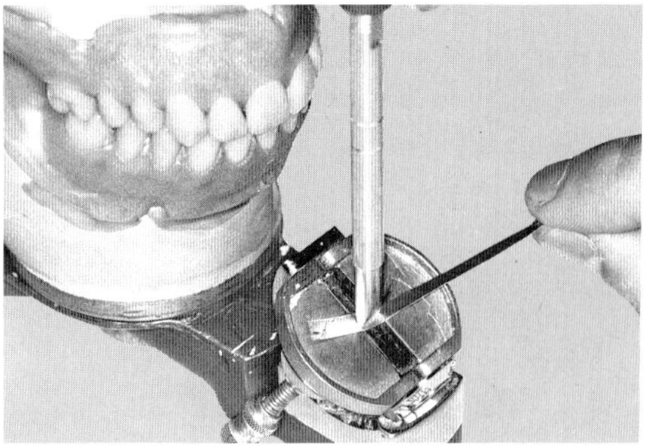

Fig. 10-1 The incisal guide table is adjusted so that the incisal guide pin stays on the guide table during protrusive and lateral movements.

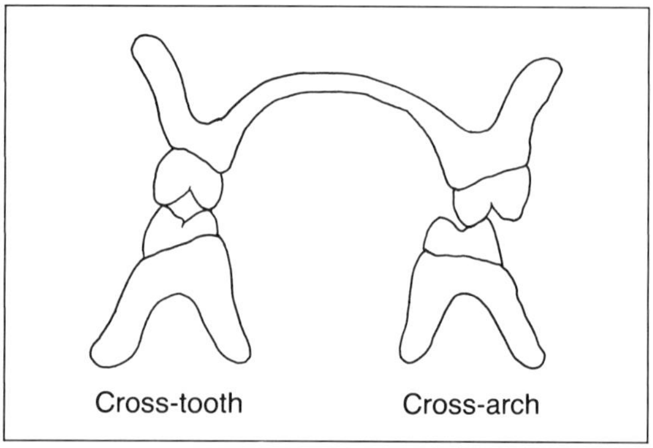

Fig. 10-2 Cross-tooth, cross-arch balance of an occlusal scheme.

Graser has shown that upon free closure with the head in an upright position, there is still some slight variation in jaw closure, anteroposteriorly as well as mediolaterally.[7] Therefore, if we desire bilateral contact in these various jaw closure positions, a balanced occlusion is necessary.

Following the initial try-in of the anterior teeth, additional information is obtained that will allow for a more objective and accurate selection of posterior teeth. A protrusive record is made (chapter 9) to provide information so that the condylar inclination can be set on the articulator. After establishing the anterior tooth positions on the patient using esthetic and phonetic guidelines, the incisal guidance is established and the incisal guide table of the articulator set accordingly (Fig. 10-1).

Prior to arranging any posterior denture teeth, a decision must be made as to whether balance is desired in the occlusal scheme. *Balance* has been defined and interpreted in many ways. The *Glossary of Prosthodontic Terms* defines it as an occlusion of the teeth which presents a harmonious relation of the occluding surfaces in all centric and eccentric positions within the functional range of mastication and swallowing.[8] The most complete form of balance is called *cross-tooth, cross-arch balance*. This means there is simultaneous contact of all the following surfaces: buccal cusps of maxillary teeth with buccal cusps of mandibular teeth, and lingual cusps of maxillary teeth with lingual cusps of mandibular teeth on the working side; lingual cusps of maxillary teeth with buccal cusps of the mandibular teeth on the balancing side (Fig. 10-2). If cross-tooth, cross-arch balance is not desired, the amount and location of the balance should be decided upon rather than waiting until insertion day to see how the teeth function in the mouth.

The incisal guide table is set so that the incisal guide pin stays on it during all eccentric movements. Esthetics and phonetics may have to be compromised to achieve an appropriate incisal guidance so that balance can be achieved in the occlusal scheme (if desired). The two end-controlling factors that will affect the cusp height needed to achieve a balanced occlusion are the incisal guidance and the condylar inclination (Fig. 10-3). Additional factors that influence the ability to achieve balance are the plane of occlusion, the compensating curve (curve of Spee), and the height and inclination of the cusps. Combined, the five factors are called the Hanau Quint or the Laws of Balanced Articulation.

After setting the anterior denture teeth for esthetics and phonetics, the amount of vertical and horizontal overlap between them can be assessed. The greater the vertical overlap and the smaller the horizontal overjet, the greater the incisal guidance will be; therefore, a steeper cusp height would be necessary to achieve a balanced occlusion (Fig. 10-4). The smaller the vertical overlap and the greater the horizontal overjet, the

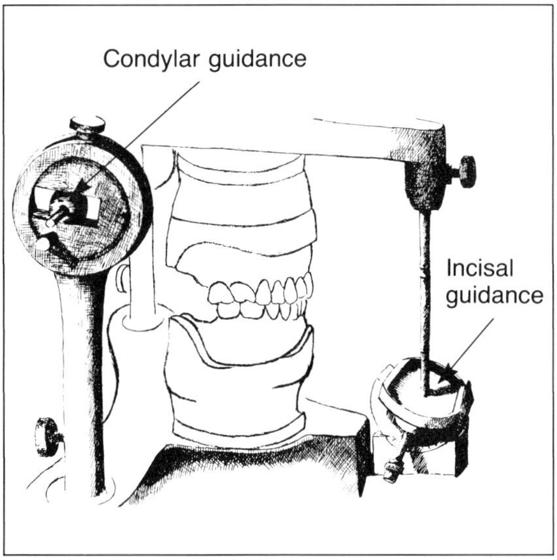

Fig. 10-3 The incisal guidance and the condylar inclination are the two end-controlling factors that guide the teeth during eccentric movement.

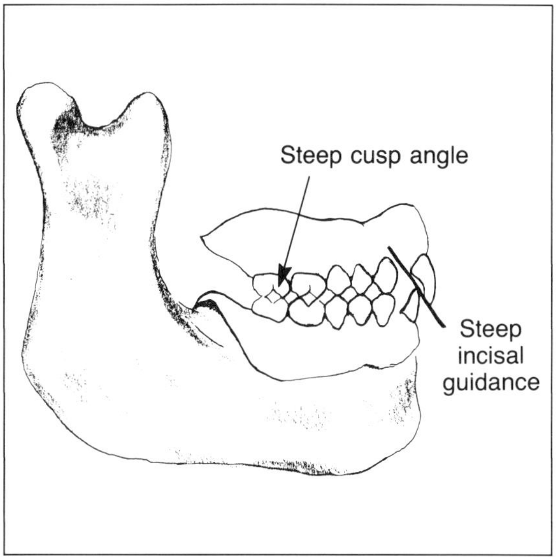

Fig. 10-4 The greater the incisal guidance angle, the steeper the cusp height needed on the posterior teeth to achieve a balanced occlusion.

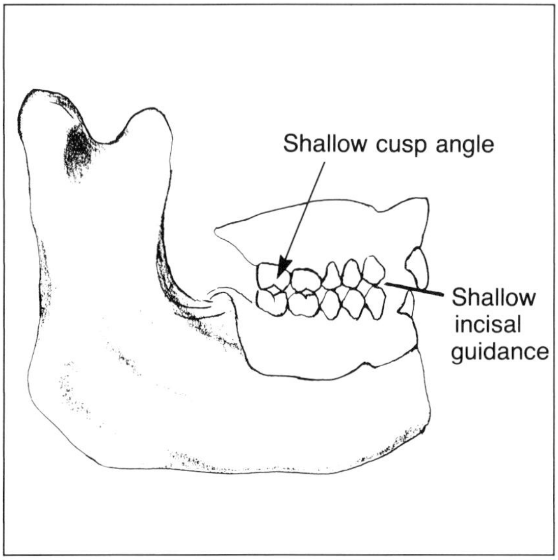

Fig. 10-5 The smaller the incisal guidance angle, the less need for a steeper cusp height to achieve balance.

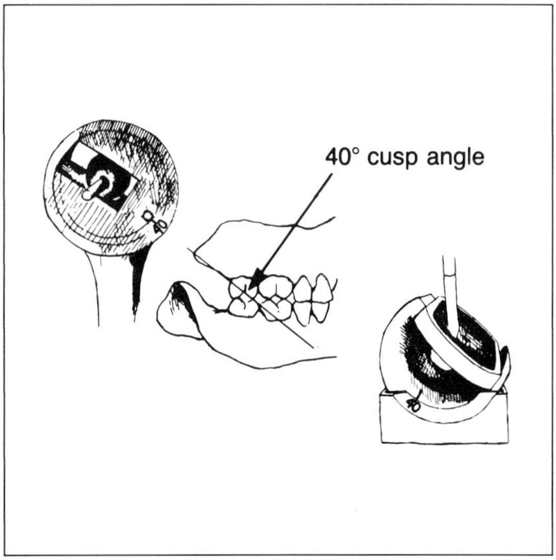

Fig. 10-6 The condylar inclination and the incisal guidance affect the degree of posterior tooth needed if balance is desired. A condylar inclination of 40° and an incisal guidance of 40° would require a posterior tooth with approximately a 40° inclination.

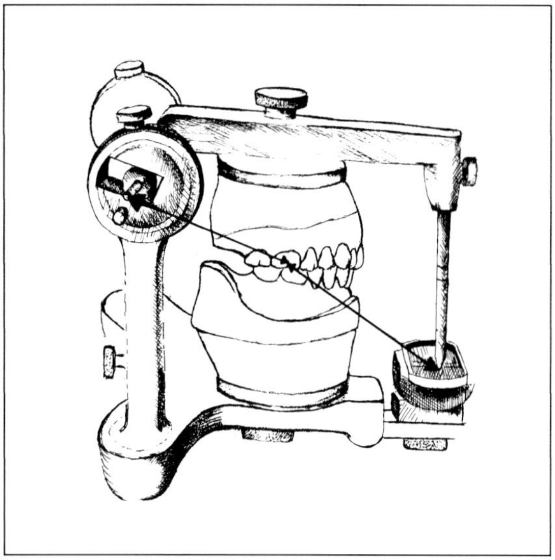

Fig. 10-7 On the articulator, the first molar is approximately equidistant from the end-controlling factors (incisal guidance and condylar inclination).

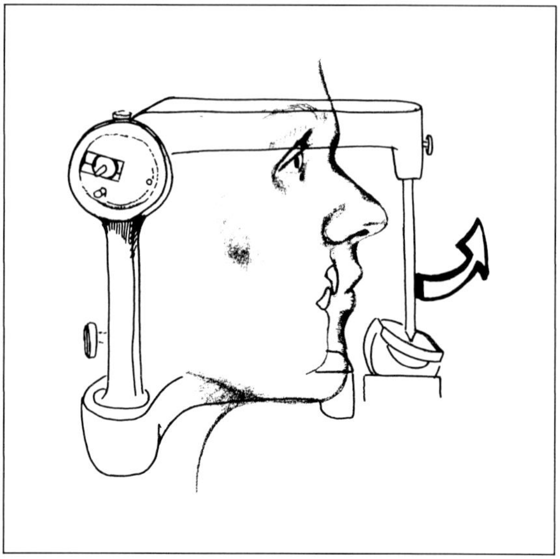

Fig. 10-8 The incisal guidance in the mouth becomes the teeth, not the incisal guide pin, and these teeth are closer to the first molar than the condylar guidance.

less need for a steeper cusp height to achieve a balanced occlusion (Fig. 10-5).

The degree of condylar inclination relative to the plane of occlusion also affects the steepness or degree of tooth needed posteriorly to achieve balance. For example, a condylar inclination that is 40° rather than 15° would require a posterior tooth of greater cusp height and angulation (Fig. 10-6).

On the articulator, the first molar is approximately equidistant from each end-controlling factor, the condylar guidance and the incisal guidance (Fig. 10-7). Therefore, the cusp height needed to achieve balance in lateral and protrusive excursions can be thought of in a mathematical or a mechanical way. For example, should the incisal guidance be 10° and the condylar guidance be 30°, the cusp height needed to balance the occlusion in the first molar region would be 20° because the first molar is mechanically halfway between the end-controlling factors (10° + 30° = 40° ÷ 2 = 20°). This is how setting the posterior denture teeth for a balanced occlusion becomes a mechanical and a mathematical problem.

In the mouth, the condylar inclination becomes a greater distance from the first molar teeth than does the incisal guidance, because the incisal guide pin is not present and the anterior denture teeth become the incisal guidance (Fig. 10-8). Therefore, the incisal guidance in the mouth will play the dominant mechanical role in determining how the posterior teeth will occlude in eccentric movements because of its relative proximity compared to the condylar inclination.

Anatomic teeth have cusp height and angulation that nonanatomic teeth do not have. If the end-controlling factors of condylar inclination and incisal guidance are steep (particularly the incisal guidance, because of its proximity to the posterior dentition), then an anatomic tooth should be considered if balance is desired. Anatomic teeth are available in varying cusp heights and angulations, and one should be selected that will fulfill the mechanical goals described. Nonanatomic posterior teeth can also be used to achieve balance if the incisal guidance is less than approximately 10°. The nonanatomic teeth are arranged to have effective cusp height by altering the plane of occlusion, the compensating curve, and the height or inclination of the teeth.

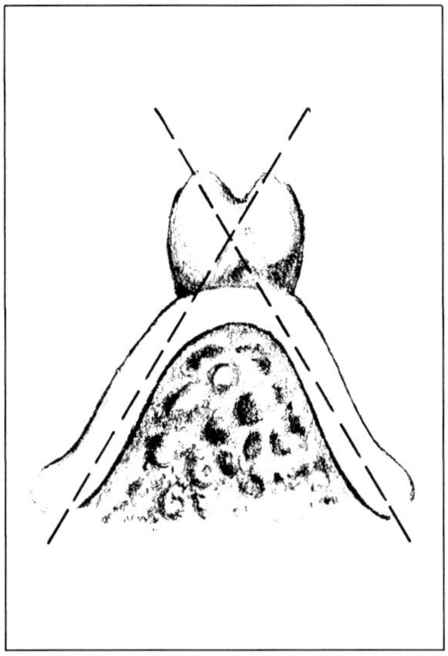

Fig. 10-9 *(left)* A well-formed ridge can accept an anatomic tooth with an angulation that conforms to the angulation of the ridge.

Fig. 10-10 *(below)* A flat ridge with a tooth that is flat to conform to it.

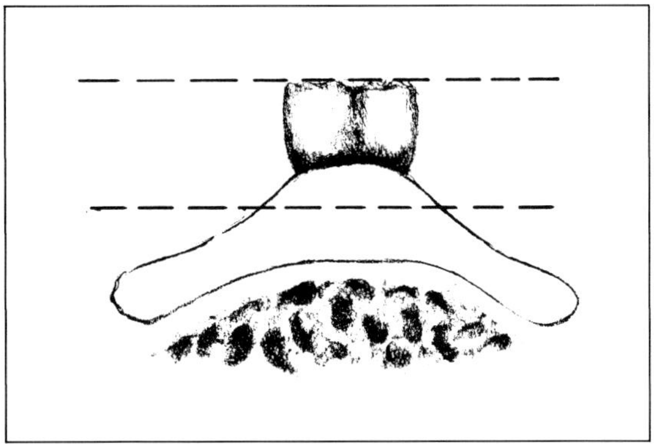

Patient age and neuromuscular coordination

Some patients experience a decrease in neuromuscular coordination as they reach their seventies and eighties. In these situations, nonanatomic posterior teeth may be preferable because they offer occlusal freedom of movement by not locking the teeth into any occlusal position. Conversely, there are many patients whose chronologic age and biologic age do not coincide (see chapter 1); for example, the patient in his seventies who looks and functions like someone in his fifties. The use of anatomic teeth in such a case may be no problem, and other criteria would have to be considered. The opposite can also be true: a 50-year-old patient with Parkinson's disease may have significant loss of neuromuscular control, and nonanatomic teeth would be indicated.

Maxillomandibular relationships

The relationship of the mandible to the maxilla in both centric jaw relation and centric occlusion is significant. The Angle's Class I occlusion patient could have either anatomic or nonanatomic teeth, depending on the other factors discussed. The Angle's Class II occlusion patient may have a large discrepancy between his centric jaw relation position and his habitual centric occlusion (see chapter 8). If a large discrepancy exists between the two positions, the patient may do better with a nonanatomic tooth form. This would give this patient the freedom to move forward or laterally from his centric jaw relation position to his centric occlusion position. An anatomic tooth set in maximum intercuspation to the centric jaw relation position may not do because the patient would be likely to function anterior to that position. The Angle's Class III occlusion patient may have a mandible that is much wider than the maxilla, resulting in a crossbite. The use of nonanatomic denture teeth allows these abnormal jaw relations to be more easily accommodated.

Reduction of the residual ridges

No definitive work has shown that anatomic or nonanatomic denture teeth preserve the residual ridge. Payne and Ortman developed criteria for posterior tooth selection based on the amount and shape of the residual ridge.[9,10] A well-formed ridge could accept an anatomic tooth form of an angulation that conformed to the angulation of the ridge (Fig. 10-9). A flat ridge, according to Ortman, could receive a flat tooth (Fig. 10-10). During years of denture wearing, Ortman states, a patient may start out with a cusped-position tooth form that in successive sets of dentures would be modified to become increasingly flatter until a flat form would be worn. The rationale for this is to decrease the lateral forces that come with age so that a compromise is reached between the efficiency of the cusps and the stability of the flat teeth, all within the tissue tolerance of the patient. This procedure is based upon subjective reasoning, however, not scientific evaluation.

Patient preference

Do patients even know if they have anatomic or nonanatomic teeth in their mouths? One study that evaluated this question used 25 subjects. Two sets of dentures were made for each.[1] One set had nonanatomic teeth, the other anatomic teeth, and subjects were not told that two different sets of dentures were being made for them. The dentures were interchanged over a period of months. None of the subjects ever knew they had two sets of dentures, and when told, all expressed disbelief. They then interchanged the dentures on their own to see if they had a preference. The results were that two preferred the anatomic posteriors, 11 preferred the nonanatomic posteriors, and ten had no preference. Two subjects did not complete the study. The reasons given for preferring the nonanatomic teeth included: "just feel better"; "look, feel, work better"; "smoother"; "speak and chew better"; "teeth not so high"; and "more comfortable and more room." The two subjects who preferred the anatomic teeth said they "look better" and "chew better." Therefore, both tooth forms were seen as suitable, and among those subjects having a preference, the nonanatomic teeth were preferred.

A second study compared lingualized occlusion and monoplane occlusion on 30 patients.[11] Of the patients, 67% preferred the lingualized occlusal scheme because of improved masticatory ability, comfort, and esthetics.

Woelfel, Hickey, and Allison compared 0°, 20°, and 33° posterior teeth on six subjects, using interchangeable posterior tooth sections.[12] Patient preference was equally divided.

Summary of advantages and indications for anatomic and nonanatomic teeth

Anatomic

The advantages of the anatomic tooth forms are their more natural appearance, greater ease in balancing occlusion, and a feeling of better chewing efficiency. Therefore, the major indications for their use are: to maximize esthetics, to provide a balanced occlusion with greater ease, to accommodate patients with good neuromuscular control, and to provide better initial penetration of the bolus.

Nonanatomic

The advantages of the nonanatomic tooth forms are that they are easier to arrange for crossbite relationships and that they give the patient the freedom to move his mandible into different jaw relationships. The major indications for using this tooth form are for patients with crossbite tooth relationships, patients with poor neuromuscular control, patients with severely resorbed ridges, and patients who have a large discrepancy between centric jaw relation and centric occlusion.

Occlusal plane and arch form

The appropriate plane of occlusion is determined by *(1)* esthetics, *(2)* occlusal function (as a factor of the Hanau Quint), and *(3)* intraoral functional factors. Esthetics is important because the posterior teeth should not appear to be too high or too low. For example, when the maxillary posterior teeth are too low, the dentures may appear as if they are falling out of the mouth when they really are not (Fig. 10-11). The occlusal plane should be level from one side of the arch to the other. If the teeth are higher on one side of the arch, an unesthetic appearance can result (Fig. 10-12).

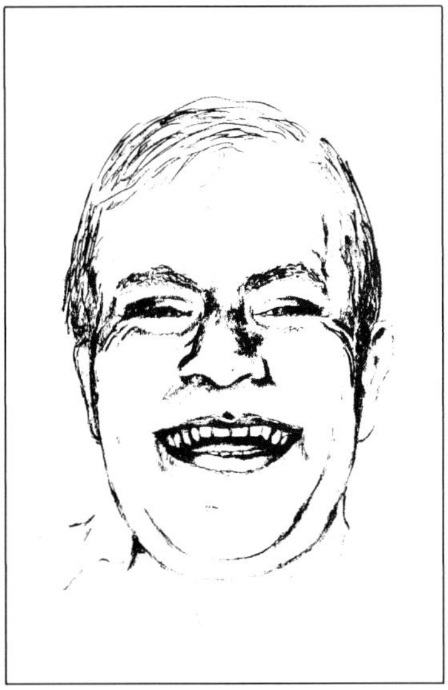

Fig. 10-11 When maxillary posterior teeth are too low they may appear unesthetic.

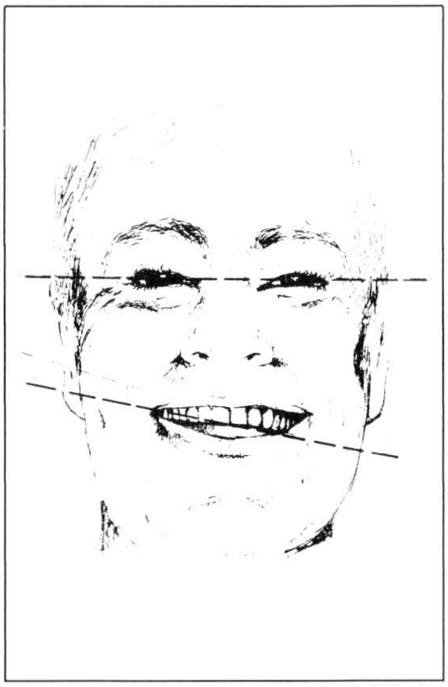

Fig. 10-12 The teeth are set higher on the right side; this should be corrected.

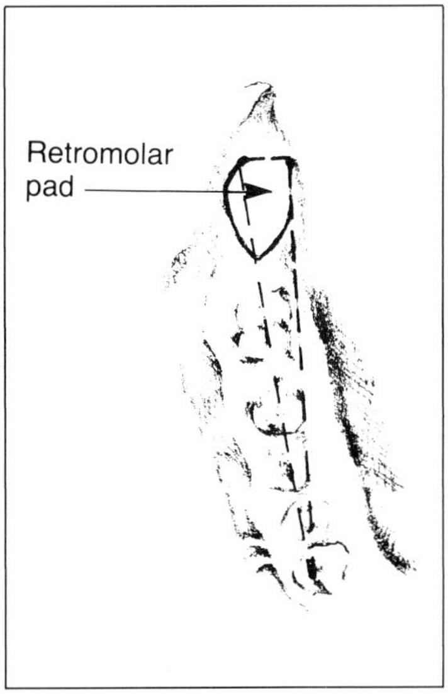

Fig. 10-13 The lingual cusps of the mandibular posterior teeth can be placed within a triangle formed by the mesial aspect of the mandibular canine and the central and lingual aspects of the retromolar pad.

The pitch of the occlusal plane is also important to increase the cusp height of the posterior denture teeth to balance the occlusion. The plane of occlusion is a factor of the Hanau Quint, as discussed earlier in this chapter. The last major consideration for the occlusal plane is intraoral factors, mainly the occlusal plane's relation to the tongue and cheeks. The plane should be at an appropriate level so that the tongue can conveniently move food onto and around the occlusal table. If the plane of occlusion is too high, it could be difficult for the tongue to shift food upon it, thereby making mastication more difficult.

Rules such as placing the central fossae over the center of the mandibular ridge often do not apply due to the amount and direction of ridge resorption. In some situations when posterior denture teeth are placed over the "center of the ridge," a too-constricted arch form can occur. The posterior teeth do not show very much when the patient smiles.

It is also important not to crowd the tongue by placing the teeth too far to the lingual. This can lead to instability of the mandibular dentures and to patient discomfort. Placing the lingual cusps within the triangular area shown in Fig. 10-13 is a reasonable guide and a good place to begin.

Anatomic tooth arrangement

The technique for arrangement of an anatomic tooth form *regardless of its degree* will now be described. Some of the important considerations will be highlighted and illustrated, but not in the form of a tooth-by-tooth demonstration, because the techniques are well illustrated in other textbooks.

1. Set the incisal guide pin to contact the incisal guide table in all eccentric movements. If the pin jumps off the table in any movement, correct this by moving the offending tooth or by grinding it. Use the guide table as a controlling factor to ensure that while each posterior tooth is being set, it is

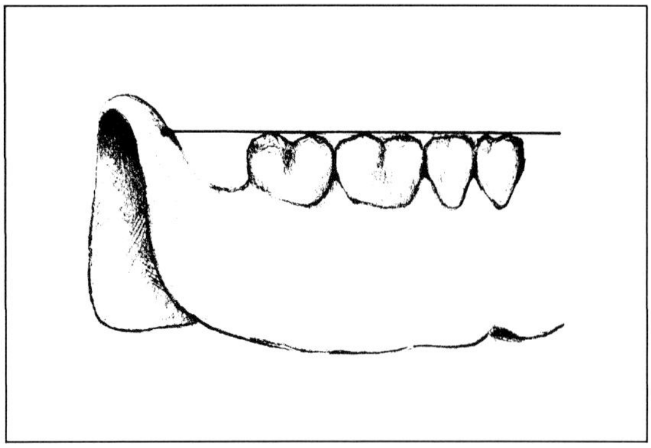

Fig. 10-14 The height of the occlusal plane should be one half to two thirds the height of the retromolar pad.

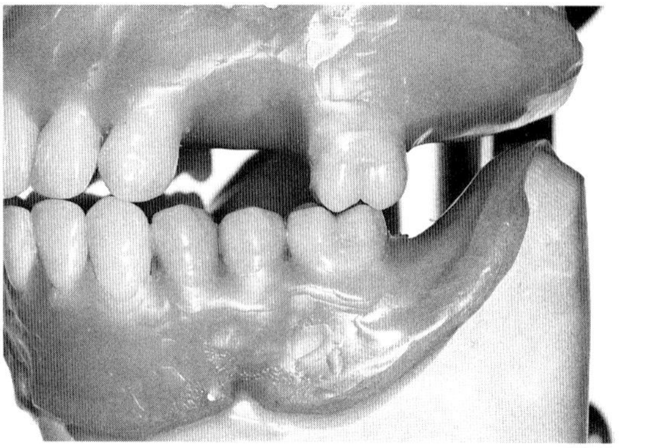

Fig. 10-15 The buccal cusps of the maxillary first molar should articulate with the mandibular first molar in the working position.

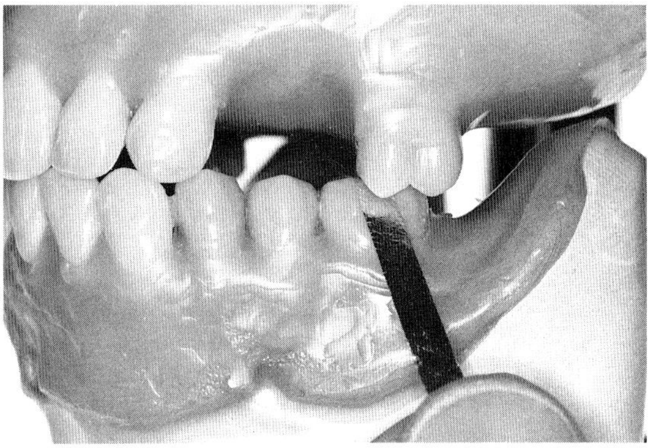

Fig. 10-16 Cut thin strips of occlusal registration material to verify that the teeth are in contact where needed.

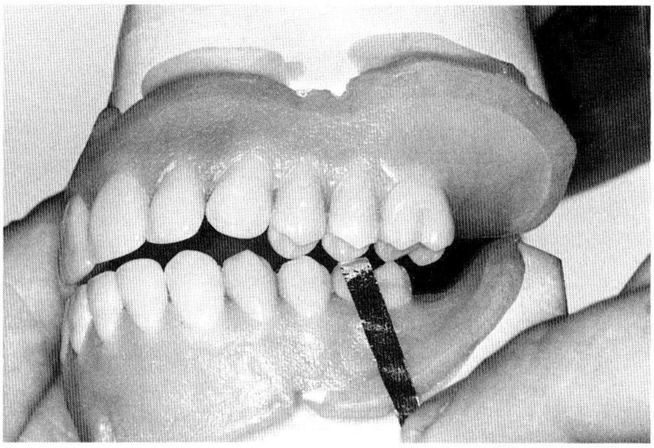

Fig. 10-17 Cross-arch balance is accomplished.

not changing the occlusion (centric or eccentric) that has been established. Use a thin piece of articulating paper or an Artus* occlusal registration strip (13-μm thickness) beneath the incisal guide pin, and pull on it to see whether the guide pin is touching the table.

2. Adapt softened baseplate wax to the mandibular posterior edentulous areas, and set up the posterior anatomic teeth bilaterally. Use the mandibular canine and the retromolar pads as guides to the superior-inferior height of the plane of occlusion. The height of the occlusal plane posteriorly should be up to one half to two thirds the height of the retromolar pad (Fig. 10-14). The mandibular lingual cusps should fall roughly within the triangle described earlier.

3. Place the maxillary first molar in a position of maximum intercuspation with the mandibular molar. When the articulator is moved into a working position, the buccal cusps of the maxillary and mandibular molars should uniformly contact, with the incisal guide pin touching the incisal guide table at the same time (Fig. 10-15). This working position is achieved to the height of the cusps as the articulator is shifted into a lateral excursion until the canines on that side are edge to edge. The lingual cusps should also have uniform con-

*Artus Co., Englewood, N.J.

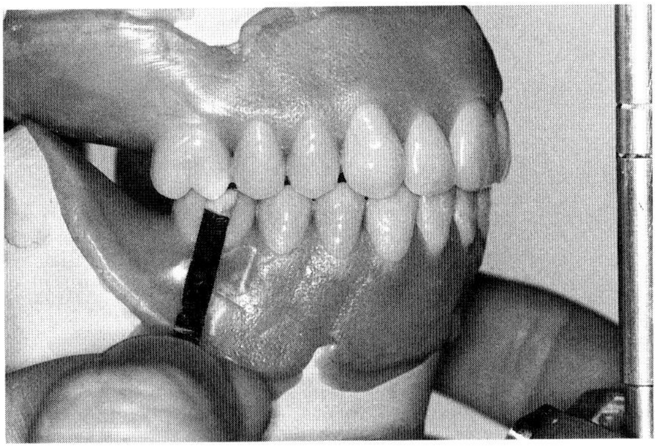

Fig. 10-18a Completed setup in centric occlusion.

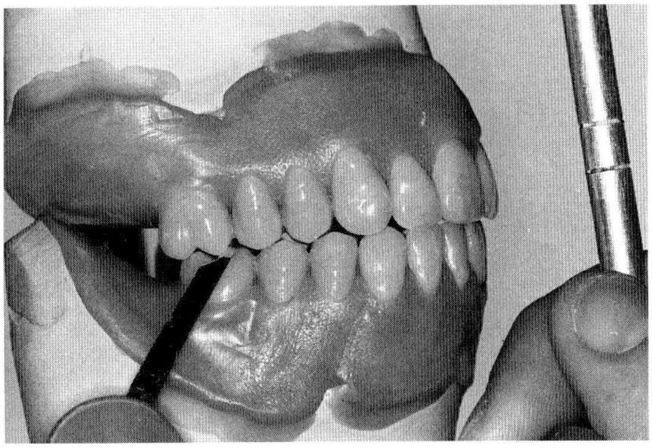

Fig. 10-18b Completed setup in working occlusion.

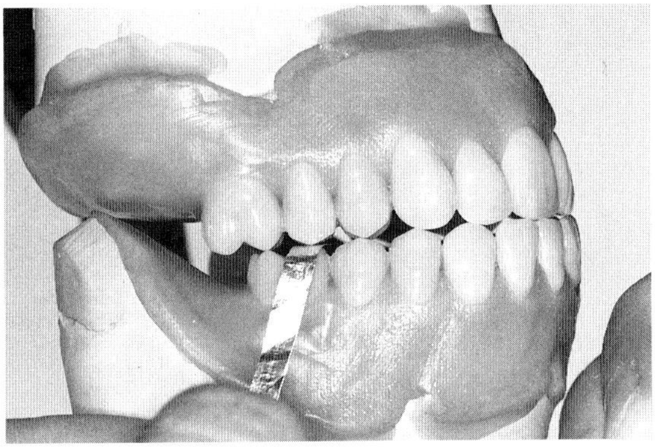

Fig. 10-18c Completed setup in protrusive occlusion.

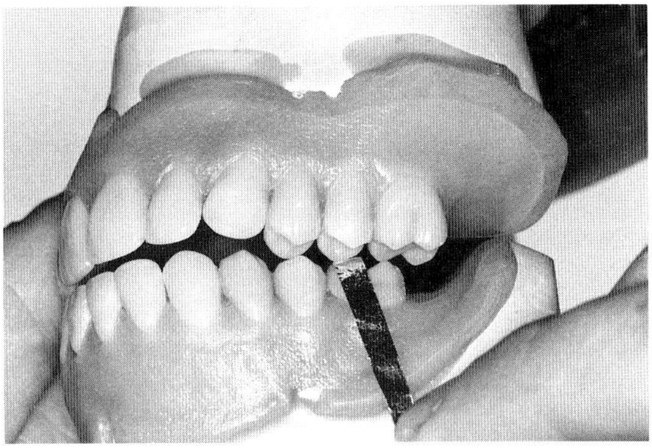

Fig. 10-18d Completed setup in balanced (cross-arch) occlusion.

tact to provide cross-tooth balance. Next, make a protrusive movement and position and adjust the teeth so that the distal aspects of the maxillary mesial cusps slide against the mesial surfaces of the mandibular distal cusps. The extent of protrusive movement is normally to position the anterior teeth edge to edge. The incisal guide pin should touch the incisal guide table in centric position and during all eccentric movements. It may be necessary first to set each maxillary posterior tooth to be "high" in centric position (the incisal pin would be off the guide table) to achieve appropriate cusp heights for a balanced occlusion.

4. Use articulating paper to mark the tooth areas that are interfering, and grind the teeth accordingly until the incisal guide pin touches the incisal guide table. Each tooth must be completely arranged and balanced before proceeding to the next. Each tooth must have appropriate contact in centric, working, protrusive, and balancing positions. Use thin articulating paper (or the Artus registration strips) cut into thin strips (2 mm wide) to test the intensity of tooth contact (Fig. 10-16). After the maxillary first molar is set, arrange the remaining maxillary teeth in the same manner beginning with the second premolar. Once one side is completely set, proceed to the opposite side and follow the same procedure. Make sure that when the articulator is moved into a working position, the teeth on the opposite side are in contact (balance). This provides for cross-

arch balance (Fig. 10-17). The mandibular teeth may have to be repositioned to alter the plane of occlusion, the compensating curve, or the height and inclination of the cusps. Make the required mandibular tooth position changes while setting each maxillary tooth. It is in this way that the teeth are positioned so as to mechanically achieve the appropriate occlusion and balance (Figs. 10-18a to d).

Nonanatomic tooth arrangement

The nonanatomic denture teeth can be arranged in the following ways:

1. Rising (or curved) occlusal plane to achieve balance
2. Monoplane concept which may negate all balance
3. Flat occlusal plane (or monoplane) with a balancing ramp

Each arrangement differs in philosophy and technique and bears some mention.

Rising (or curved) occlusal plane to achieve balance

In this situation, the factors of the Hanau Quint are used to achieve balance in the occlusion or to achieve the working occlusion desired. If a particular patient has a significant discrepancy between the centric jaw relation position and the centric occlusion position (or neuromuscular position), the patient may close habitually into the centric occlusion position. As described in chapter 9, this discrepancy may be several millimeters or more. If a centric jaw relation record was made to mount the mandibular denture, the patient may not have maximum intercuspation in the centric occlusion position because it is anterior to the centric jaw relation position. Therefore, to provide maximum occlusion in the centric occlusion position, a protrusive balance must be built into the occlusal scheme. The incisal guidance, the plane of occlusion, and the height and inclination of the teeth would have to be adjusted (Fig. 10-19). (The Hanau No. 2 articulator is a rectilinear articulator—it moves in straight lines—therefore a compensating curve cannot be arranged upon it.)

Monoplane concept which may negate all balance

With the monoplane concept, the teeth are arranged so that they are on a single plane parallel to the floor. The teeth are set and the articulator is programmed to negate *all* factors of the Hanau Quint (Fig. 10-20). No rising plane of occlusion is developed, and the teeth are set to have no cusp height or inclination. Without these factors there is no way to achieve balance in excursive movements.

Flat occlusal plane (or monoplane) with a balancing ramp

In this occlusal scheme, balance is achieved by altering the cusp height and angulation of the first or second molar (Fig. 10-21). This is accomplished by tilting the distal portion of the molar higher than the occlusal plane of the other posterior teeth. When a patient moves into protrusive or working position, the tilted molar (ramp) will make contact, and what the proponents of this technique call "balance" will be achieved.

The arrangement of the nonanatomic teeth with a rising flat occlusal plane will now be described. Set the articulator in the same manner as for the arrangement of the anatomic teeth. Then follow these steps:

1. Set the mandibular posterior teeth so that the occlusal surfaces are on a rising flat plane from the incisal edge of the canine to approximately one half to two thirds up the retromolar pad. If balance is desired in the occlusal scheme, the incisal guidance must be kept to below 10°. Set them buccolingually so that the center of the fossae is in line with the tip of the canine and the center of the retromolar pad.
2. Set the maxillary first molar in centric po-

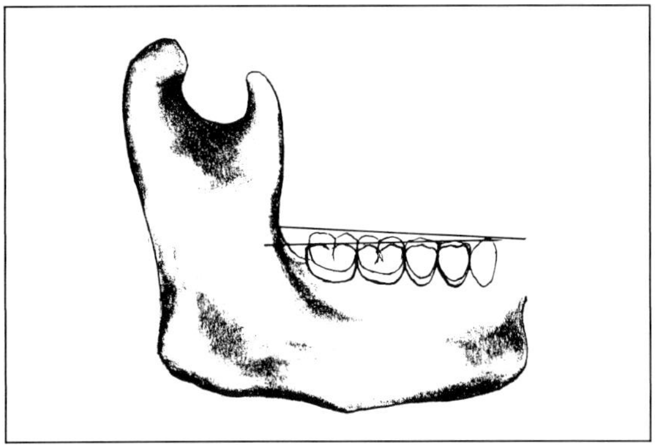

Fig. 10-19 The plane of occlusion is made to rise posteriorly to help achieve protrusive balance.

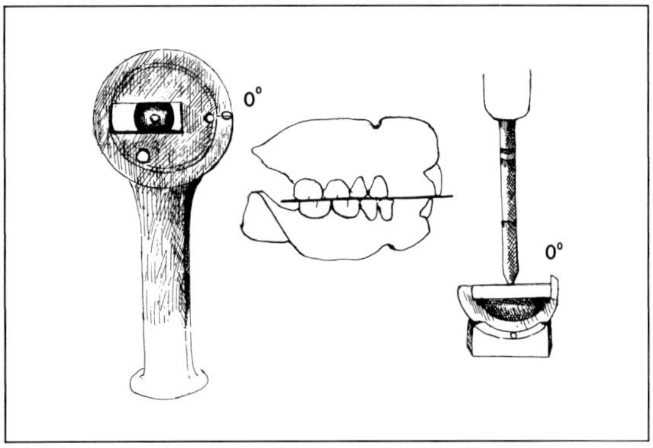

Fig. 10-20 In the monoplane concept, there is no rise to the plane of occlusion posteriorly. No protrusive balance is achieved.

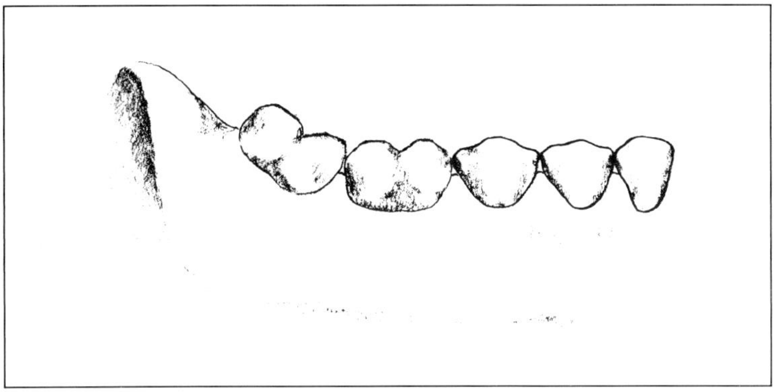

Fig. 10-21 A balancing ramp is provided for by using an exaggerated tilt on the first or second molars. Balance is provided at the most distal portion of the ramp.

sition. Position the tooth so as to achieve working and balancing contact. As with anatomic teeth, it is sometimes necessary to move the mandibular teeth (to change the pitch of the teeth) or to set the tooth to be high in centric position. If the tooth is set high in centric position, grind the tooth in eccentric and finally centric positions.

3. Now set the maxillary second premolar so as to make contact in centric jaw relation, followed by contact in working and nonworking lateral movements. If contact is not achieved in these lateral movements, the tooth may again need to be set high in the centric position and then spot ground in the lateral movements.

4. Set the maxillary first premolar in the same manner just described for the other maxillary teeth. If space exists between the canine and the first premolar, it can be very helpful in providing a more natural appearance. If the distance is too great, space can be left between the first and second premolar, as well as between the canine and first premolar.

5. Finally, the second molar is positioned in a similar manner when there is sufficient space. All 16 posterior teeth do not always have to be set on the dentures. Occasionally, the second molar or second premolar may be omitted when the total length of the posterior teeth exceeds the denture space available. This would be evident when the last mandibular posterior tooth would sit in a position resting upon the retromolar pad. This is a situation which could lead to denture instability.

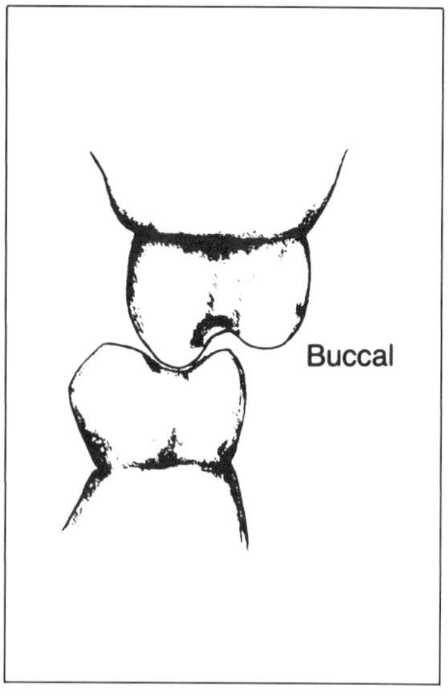

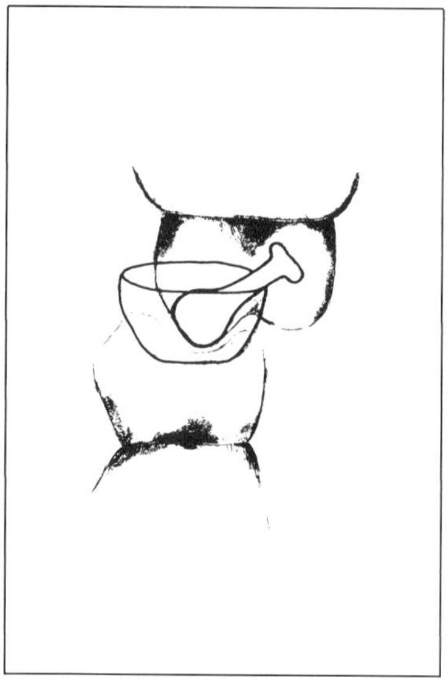

Fig. 10-22 *(left)* The maxillary lingual cusp functions against the mandibular teeth in all excursions, hence the term lingualized occlusion.

Fig. 10-23 *(right)* Lingualized occlusion is compared to the use of a mortar and pestle.

Lingual cusp occlusion

Lingual cusp occlusion occurs when the maxillary lingual cusp opposes a mandibular occlusal surface as the only centric holding cusp. The maxillary lingual cusp is the only cusp that functions in eccentric movements. This type of occlusal scheme is a compromise between an anatomic and nonanatomic occlusal scheme. Usually maxillary anatomic teeth (30° to 33° teeth) are selected to oppose mandibular nonanatomic teeth (0°) for a lingualized occlusion. A functional posterior anatomic tooth with shallow cusps (10°) can be used for the mandibular posterior teeth. Follow these steps:

1. Arrange the mandibular posterior teeth as previously described for the nonanatomic tooth setup.
2. Cut a slight groove, or trough, down the center of the mandibular occlusal surface or in the position where the lingual cusp of the maxilla touches the mandibular occlusal surface. Position each maxillary tooth so that the lingual cusps are set into this groove. Tilt the maxillary teeth so that the buccal cusps are raised higher than normal and will not touch the mandibular teeth in any excursions. When the patient moves into a working relationship, the lingual cusp of the maxillary tooth functions against the mandibular tooth, hence the term *lingualized occlusion* (Fig. 10-22).

This technique lends itself to the use of a raised or curved plane of occlusion when a balanced occlusion is desired. The lingualized occlusion concept allows a sharp, penetrating cusp on the maxilla to occlude against a relatively flat occlusal plane. An analogy often drawn is to compare this concept to a mortar and pestle action (Fig. 10-23). The lingual cusps of the maxillary teeth are free to move in all directions easily; therefore, they have the advantage of the use of nonanatomic teeth with the added benefit of sharp, penetrating cusps. The patient is not "locked into" a centric position, as might be the case with anatomic teeth.

Summary

The use of only one type of posterior tooth form, anatomic or nonanatomic, for all patients is an oversimplification. There are advantages and indications for each type, and at times the two forms may be used in combination. Conversely, there are disadvantages and contraindications for each.

Although the technician may be primarily responsible for setting the posterior teeth, it is the dentist's responsibility to select the proper teeth and to determine whether they have been set correctly and balanced adequately. Simultaneous contact on both sides upon initial closure is very important, but because the jaw may close in different positions depending upon the posture of the head, a balanced occlusion will allow for uniform contact in these various positions.

References

1. Brewer, A.A., Reibel, P.R., and Nassif, N.J. Comparison of zero-degree and anatomic teeth on complete dentures. J. Prosthet. Dent. 17:28, 1967.
2. Hickey, J.C., Henderson, D., and Straus, R. Patient response to variations in denture technique. Part I. Design of a study. J. Prosthet. Dent. 22:158, 1969.
3. Nichol, B., et al. Patient response to variations in denture technique. Part II. Five year cephalometric evaluation. J. Prosthet. Dent. 41:368, 1979.
4. Ellinger, C., et al. Patient response to variations in denture technique. Part III. Five year subjective evaluation. J. Prosthet. Dent. 42:127, 1979.
5. Brehm, T.W., and Abadi, B.J. Patient response to variations in complete denture technique. Part IV. Residual ridge resorption—cast evaluation. J. Prosthet. Dent. 44:491–494, 1980.
6. Sabes, W.R., et al. Patient response to variations in denture technique. Part V. Microscopic response of the oral mucosa. J. Prosthet. Dent. 45:11–13, 1981.
7. Graser, G.N. Terminal hinge position or neuromuscular position: an evaluation of the edentulous. Part I. Maxillomandibular recordings. J. Prosthet. Dent. 36:491–500, 1976.
8. Academy of Denture Prosthetics. Glossary of Prosthodontic Terms. 4th ed. St. Louis: C.V. Mosby Co., 1977.
9. Payne, S.H. A posterior setup to meet individual requirements. Dent. Bk. 47:20–22, 1941.
10. Ortman, H.R. The role of occlusion in preservation and prevention in complete denture prosthodontics. J. Prosthet. Dent. 25:121–138, 1971.
11. Clough, H.E., et al. A comparison of lingualized occlusion and monoplane occlusion in complete dentures. J. Prosthet. Dent. 50:176, 1983.
12. Woelfel, J.B., Hickey, J.C., and Allison, M.L. Effect of posterior tooth form and jaw and denture movement. J. Prosthet. Dent. 12:922–939, 1962.

The history of dentistry is a history of expediency research. What we have does not work so someone makes great claims for what he has developed. Frequently these claims are based on observation of one patient or observation of many patients without comparison of the results of using a different instrument or material or denture tooth.

Procedures based on judgment, not backed up by experimentation, are always suspect. The experimentation should be performed on a comparative basis.

Allen Brewer
(Personal communication)

Chapter 11

Try-in of the Trial Denture

The try-in of the trial denture is perhaps one of the most important appointments for both the patient and the dentist. It is during this visit that the dentist and patient have the opportunity to evaluate many of the previous steps already accomplished. It is easier to make gross changes or corrections at this time rather than to wait until the dentures have been completed. Any additional time spent during this phase of treatment is usually time well spent.

The try-in of the trial denture is divided into the following clinical procedures which will be discussed separately: evaluation of the vertical dimension of occlusion, evaluation of the centric occlusion position, esthetic considerations, and patient approval.

Evaluation of the vertical dimension of occlusion

The clinical rest position

Determine whether the patient has adequate interocclusal distance with the trial dentures in the mouth. At this time you can have the patient stand up or remain seated in the dental chair. If the patient remains seated, be sure that he is in an upright position and his head is not supported by the headrest. The headrest may affect the clinical rest position of the mandible and therefore influence the amount of interocclusal distance seen. Regardless, be sure that the patient is at ease and comfortable. This is a clinical procedure that cannot be hurried. Rushing can make the patient feel anxious.

The important clinical judgment is whether, at this vertical dimension of occlusion, the patient has adequate room between his teeth when his mandible is in a clinical resting position. Instruct the patient to wet his lips, swallow, and then allow his mandible to rest. While the patient is in this resting position, part his lips to see whether his teeth are touching. Before parting the lips, caution the patient not to move any part of his mouth or jaw. If the teeth are in contact while the mandible is at rest, the vertical dimension of occlusion is too open and a new vertical dimension of occlusion should be established.

Phonetic tests

After denture teeth are set up, phonetics is the most significant guideline for evaluating the previously selected vertical dimension of occlusion. The vertical dimension of occlusion should never be accepted as correct until the patient has been put through a series of phonetic tests.

Instruct the patient to count from 50 to 60 and ask him to tell you if his teeth touch and at what numbers they touch. If the patient's teeth make contact during speech, it is usually an indication that there is not enough interocclusal distance during speech. This is why some patients' denture teeth clack during speech. Pound refers to what he

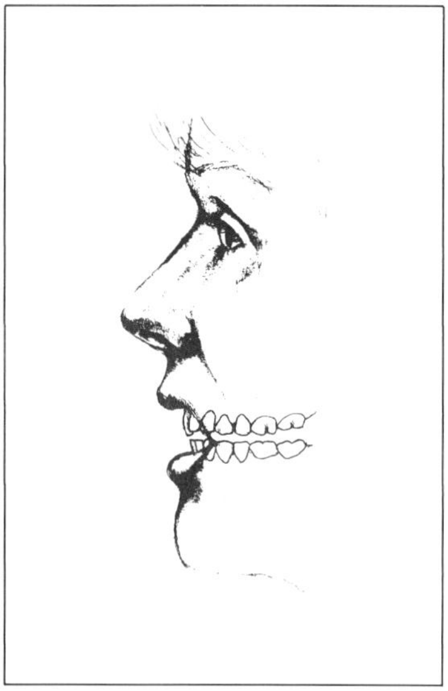

Fig. 11-1 An anterior and posterior speaking space exists between the teeth when sibilant sounds are made.

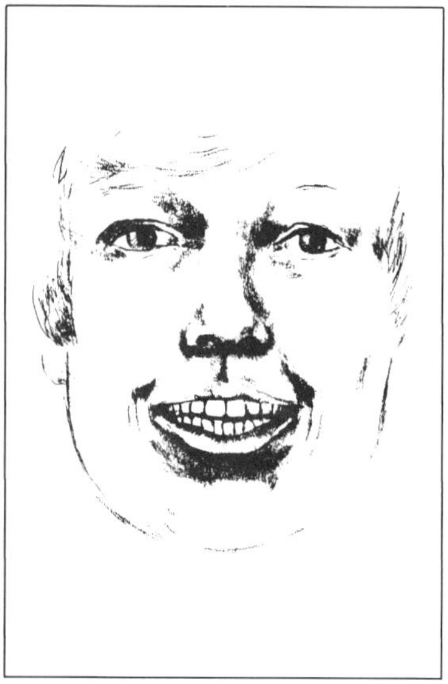

Fig. 11-2 The mandibular anterior teeth almost touch the maxillary anterior teeth when the "s" sound is articulated.

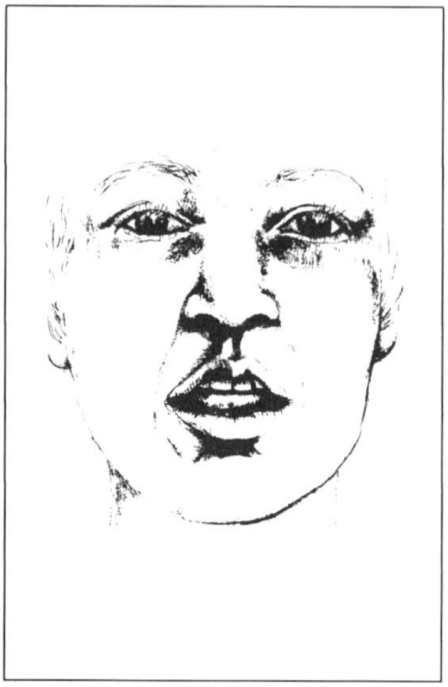

Fig. 11-3 Twenty percent of the denture-wearing population use their tongues to help articulate the "s" sound. In these patients, the anterior teeth do not closely approximate each other.

calls the "anterior speaking space" and the "posterior speaking space"; that is, the space between the anterior or posterior teeth when the patient articulates sibilant or "s" sounds[1] (Fig. 11-1).

While the patient counts from 50 to 60, pay particular attention to the "s" sounds. In most patients, during articulation of the "s" sounds, the mandibular anterior teeth move downward and forward to approach within 0.5 to 1 mm of the incisal edges of the maxillary anterior teeth—the teeth almost touch (Fig. 11-2). As the anterior teeth approach each other, the teeth and the small space between them control the flow of air and articulate the "s" sound clearly without a whistle or hiss. If a space greater than 0.5 to 1 mm exists during sibilant sounds, the vertical dimension of occlusion may need to be increased or the position of the anterior teeth changed. On the other hand, if the anterior or posterior teeth contact each other during speech, the vertical dimension of occlusion likely needs to be decreased. If only the anterior teeth contact, the anterior teeth may be positioned incorrectly.

Pound reports that approximately 20% of the denture population has what he calls an *atypical "s" sound*, in which the anterior teeth do not closely approximate each other during sibilant sounds and the tongue is used to help articulate the sounds (Fig. 11-3). Pound says that for patients with atypical "s" sounds, no matter how much you increase the vertical dimension of occlusion, the anterior teeth will still remain significantly separated when "s" sounds are made. This finding highlights the importance of using other clinical guidelines besides phonetics in assessing the patient's vertical dimension of occlusion.

Other supportive phonetic tests of the vertical dimension of occlusion include the following:

1. Have the patient say "s, s, s, s," *rapidly* and observe the anterior and posterior teeth. Perhaps the best method is to observe the patient in uninhibited conversational speech. Engage the patient in conversation or have the patient read aloud from a magazine or book.
2. Instruct the patient to pronounce the words

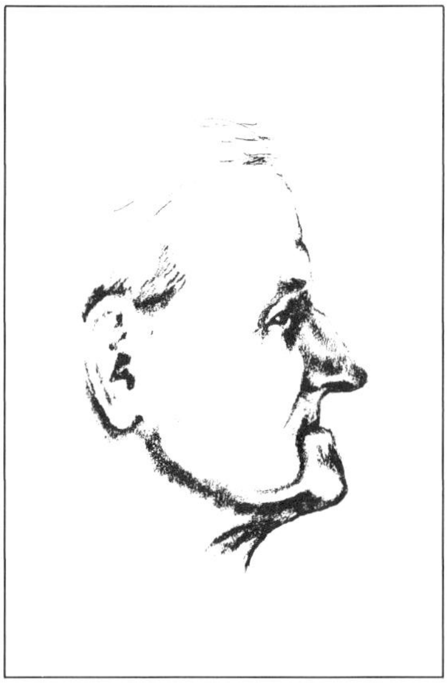

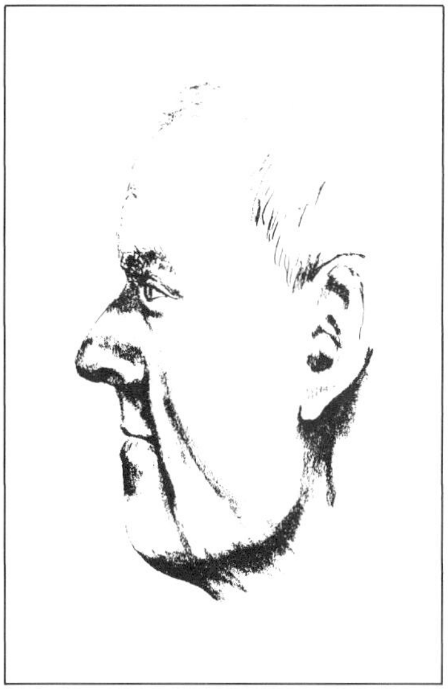

Fig. 11-4a *(left)* A patient with a decreased vertical dimension of occlusion.

Fig. 11-4b *(right)* A patient with an increased vertical dimension of occlusion.

*j*udge and *ch*urch because the "j" and "ch" sounds can be used as guides to the adequacy of the horizontal and vertical overlap of the anterior teeth. If there were inadequate room, the mandibular teeth might clash with the maxillary teeth.

3. Instruct the patient to say words with "th": *th*is, *th*at, *th*ese, *th*ose, *th*irty-*th*ree. The tongue should protrude slightly to occupy the interocclusal space between the anterior teeth.

4. Instruct the patient to pronouce the letter *m* in rapid succession. The mandible should remain relatively stationary while the lips contact each other to make the sound. Have the patient say words like "*M*ississippi" or "E*mm*a" and then have him relax his jaw to see if adequate interocclusal space exists.

Facial expression, facial form, and esthetics

Facial form is an important guide to whether the patient is at the correct vertical dimension of occlusion. Figures 11-4a and b show a profile of a patient at an overclosed (decreased) vertical dimension of occlusion and someone with an overopened (increased) vertical dimension of occlusion. Age and vertical dimension of occlusion are shown in Figs. 11-5a and b. An esthetic proportionality between the lower face height and upper face height usually exists when the patient is at the correct vertical dimension of occlusion as described by Blumenthal.[2] He suggests that dentists look carefully at the masterful art work of Leonardo da Vinci, who paid exacting attention to vertical dimension and its esthetic importance.

The degree of visibility of the maxillary and mandibular denture teeth is a helpful guideline in determining an appropriate vertical dimension of occlusion. Esthetics is often overlooked when assessing vertical dimension. It is critical to evaluate the amount and location of tooth display while the patient rests, speaks, and smiles. The more increased the vertical dimension, the more display of the maxillary and mandibular teeth, because teeth are moved to occupy more of the interocclusal space. The opposite is also true: the more decreased the vertical dimension of occlusion, the less tooth display. At the selected vertical dimension of occlusion try to achieve an esthetic and appropriate display of teeth.

Esthetic problems often occur as a result of changing a patient's vertical dimension when new dentures are made. For example, many patients present for treatment with highly worn denture teeth and increased ridge resorption under their existing dentures, which are perhaps 20 years old. Because of the tooth wear and bone loss, such a patient may not display much tooth during rest,

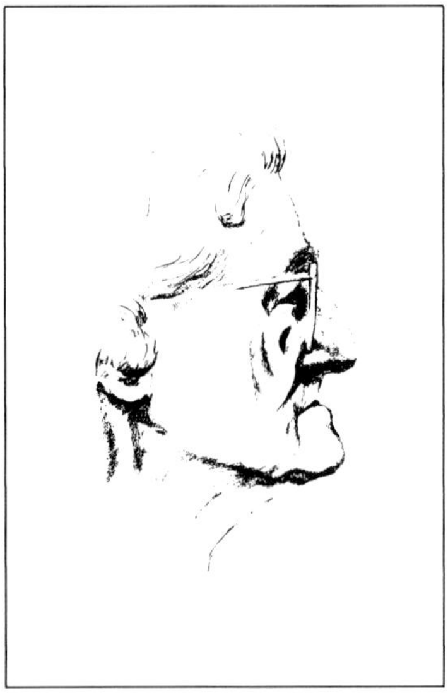

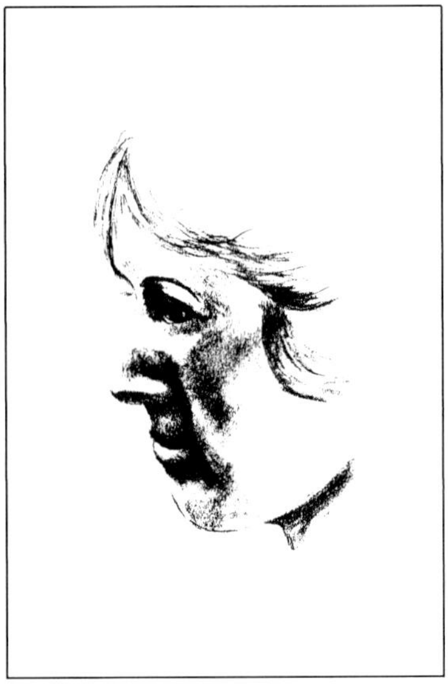

Figs. 11-5a and b Age versus youth: drawings of the same woman at ages 78 and 20.

speech, or smiling. In the making of new dentures for such a patient, we are likely to decide to increase the vertical dimension of occlusion using the criteria previously mentioned. The problem arises because at this new increased vertical dimension of occlusion, the patient will show more teeth and, therefore, look different than before. This esthetic change may be unacceptable to the patient or to the patient's family or friends. Often, it is necessary to compromise on the needed vertical opening to satisfy the patient's esthetic needs.

To conclude, never depend upon merely one or two guidelines in assessing the patient's vertical dimension. Vertical dimension cannot be thought of as an exact numerical measurement. Rather it should be thought of in terms of the clinical criteria and clinical judgments described.

Evaluation of the centric occlusion position

The second major step during the try-in visit is to evaluate the centric occlusion position or the free, unguided closure position that the patient assumes. This is the occlusal position that the patient closes into when his mandible is not guided by the operator. It is easiest and most practical to have the patient sit in the dental chair, making certain that his head is upright and not supported by the headrest. Ask the patient to open and close his mouth, and look at the teeth to see if there is even bilateral tooth contact when the teeth first touch. The centric jaw relation position was previously verified as correct by using checkpoints; we are now checking to see if the patient closes habitually anterior and/or lateral to the centric jaw relation position. It is important that the occlusion be correct at the position that the patient will close into habitually. It is best to find this out at the try-in rather than after the dentures have been inserted. If a discrepancy does exist and the occlusal contacts are not correct in the centric occlusion position, the following should be done.

1. The dentures can be balanced on the articulator so that there is maximum intercuspation in both the centric jaw relation position and the centric occlusion position. This is the reason why a protrusive record is so important. The protrusive record is used to set the condylar inclination path so that the articulator can be used to build in "protrusive" balance from the centric jaw relation position to the centric occlusion position.

2. When the discrepancy between centric jaw

relation and centric occlusion is too large (greater than 3 mm), it may be necessary to remount the dentures in the centric occlusion position. Make a centric occlusion record, and remount the mounting cast to a second mounting ring with a keyed stone index. Keep the original centric jaw relation mounting ring and the keyed stone index. Both mountings will be used to develop the occlusal scheme. Maximum intercuspation can be achieved using the centric occlusion articulation, and the centric jaw relation mounting can be used to verify that there are even tooth contacts in the centric jaw relation position.

The checkpoints were used after the centric jaw relation position was verified to see the discrepancy between the centric jaw relation position and centric occlusion position (chapter 8). Looking at this factor again when the teeth are set up is important, because the sensory mechanism of the patient may be different when teeth are set up in the mouth.

Esthetic considerations

The final step at the try-in appointment and perhaps the most challenging and difficult is the completion of the esthetic arrangement of the denture teeth. During this time it is also important to evaluate the plane of occlusion as it relates to patient esthetics and function.

Plane of occlusion

A properly oriented occlusal plane is important to patient esthetics, patient comfort and chewing function, and the balance of the occlusion. The plane of occlusion as it relates to balance of the occlusion was discussed in chapter 10. The discussion here will deal with the occlusal plane as it relates to patient function and esthetics.

Functional aspects of the plane of occlusion

If the plane of occlusion is either too high or too low in relation to the position of the tongue at rest, the patient may have problems chewing or stabilizing the mandibular denture. If the plane of occlusion is well above the tongue, the patient may have significant problems shifting food onto the food table (the occlusal surfaces of the teeth) while eating (Fig. 11-6). This can seriously impair the patient's masticatory efficiency and comfort while eating. In addition, if the occlusal plane is too elevated, the patient would find it difficult to use his tongue to move food out of the vestibules while eating. When the occlusal plane is too high, a patient may also complain that food collects readily along the borders of the mandibular denture. If the occlusal plane is too high, the tongue may not rest appropriately upon the lingual denture surfaces to assist in stabilizing the denture.

Esthetic aspects of the plane of occlusion

The most commonly used guideline to establish the plane of occlusion is Camper's line. Camper's line is a line drawn from the superior portion of the tragus of the ear to the inferior border of the ala of the nose[3] (Fig. 11-7). The occlusal plane is made parallel to this line. When Camper's line is used exclusively to determine the plane of occlusion, the maxillary denture teeth may look as if they are falling down posteriorly.

The occlusal plane can affect the way the dentures look, particularly when the patient smiles broadly. Another guideline is to orient the occlusal plane on the mandibular denture so that the posterior denture teeth rise in relationship to the retromolar pad posteriorly. Check posteriorly to see that the height of the last denture tooth is approximately one half to two thirds the height of the retromolar pad. The plane of occlusion should be the same height bilaterally. To check this, place an instrument on the posterior denture teeth on the articulator. Use a tongue blade intraorally to check whether the occlusal plane is symmetrical bilaterally in the mouth in relation to the intrapupillary line (Fig. 11-8).

Whatever methods are used to establish the occlusal plane, the final check is to determine whether the plane of occlusion is appropriate cosmetically for the patient. Look at the patient when he is at rest, speaking, and smiling.

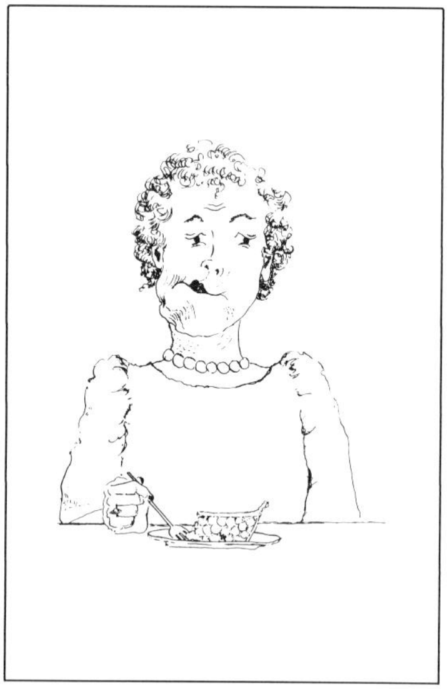

Fig. 11-6 If the occlusal plane is elevated well above the tongue, the patient may have problems shifting food onto the occlusal table.

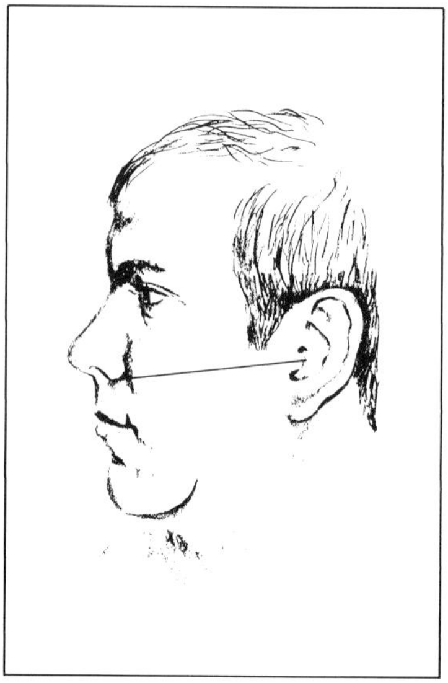

Fig. 11-7 Camper's line is a line drawn from the superior border of the tragus of the ear to the ala of the nose. The occlusal plane is made parallel to this line.

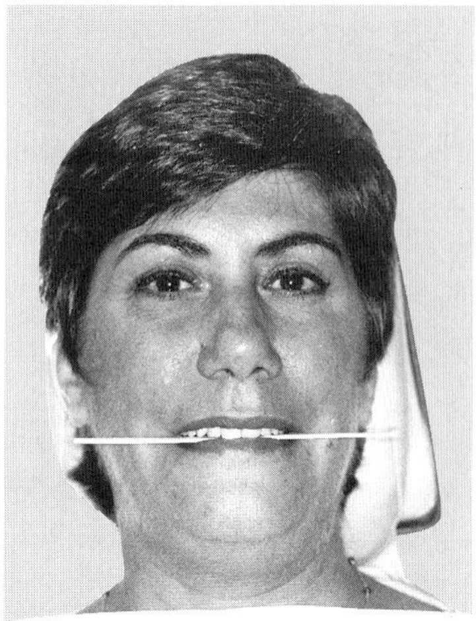

Fig. 11-8 A tongue blade is used intraorally to verify that the occlusal plane is symmetrical in the mouth in relation to the interpupillary line.

The anatomic wax-up

Complete the wax-up prior to the final esthetic check by the dentist and patient. After the patient accepts the wax-up, it is critical that neither the dentist nor the laboratory technician makes any changes to the gingival height or contour that could adversely affect the smile line and the size and shape of the teeth.

1. Flow fluid baseplate wax onto the labial and buccal surfaces using a No. 31 wax spatula (Fig. 11-9). A No. 31 spatula is used because it is large enough to carry a significant amount of wax and is the appropriate shape to fit between the teeth to form the papillae. Never flow warm wax onto the lingual surfaces at the same time; the teeth could move, because all the wax would be soft. Keep either the buccal or lingual surfaces cool to keep the teeth in their proper position.
2. Carve the wax around the gingivae of the teeth with the pointed end of a No. 7 wax spatula to create the outline form of the teeth desired (Fig. 11-10).
3. Use the angled end of a wax carver to bevel the wax toward the tooth and to clean away excess wax. The final gingival outline form is created at this time. If additional wax is needed, flow it on. The gingival outline form can change the character of the tooth shape and mold. For example, a square tooth can be made to look tapered or a tapered tooth can be contoured at the gingival portion to look square (see chapter 10).
4. Use a small vulcanite scraper or a No. 7 wax spatula to carve the available wax to create a natural-looking gingival and mucosal form (Fig. 11-11). It is sometimes necessary to add additional baseplate wax to properly develop the canine eminences and labial frena.
5. Use thin dental floss to remove excess wax between the anterior teeth (Fig. 11-12). If the wax between the teeth is not removed, acrylic resin will be processed between the teeth, leading to an unesthetic appearance or at least difficulty removing it after processing.
6. Make certain additional baseplate wax overlaps the butt joint on the completed bases. The acrylic resin shrinks during processing, and this

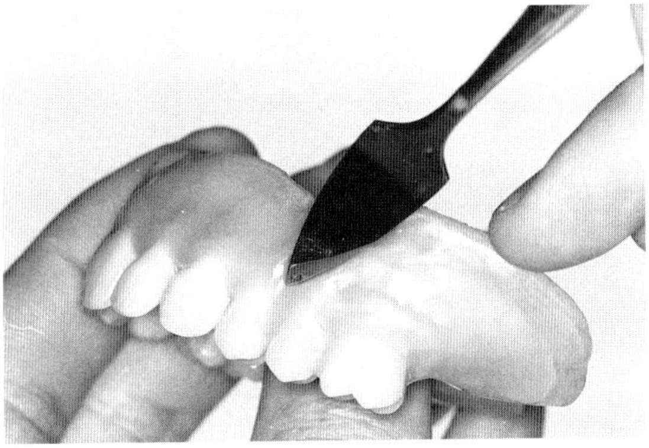

Fig. 11-9 Fluid baseplate wax is flowed onto the labial and buccal surfaces of the base.

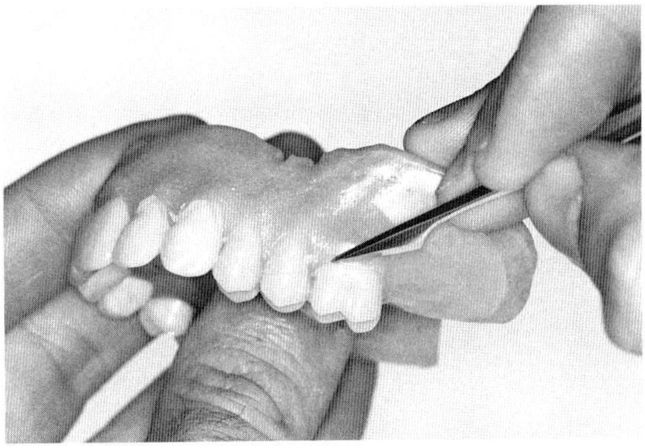

Fig. 11-10 The pointed end of a spatula is used to create the gingival form.

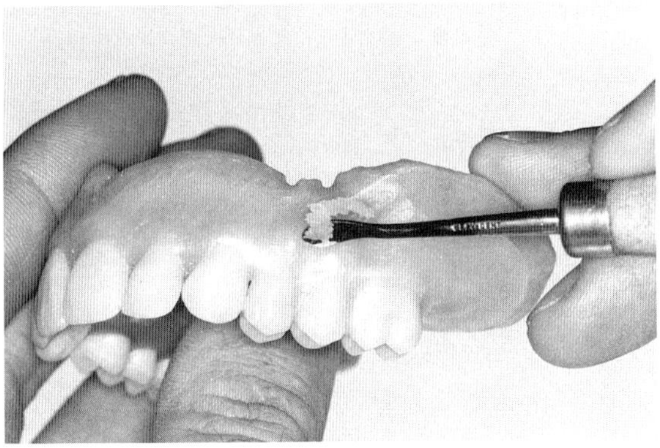

Fig. 11-11 A vulcanite scraper is used to carve the available wax to develop anatomic character.

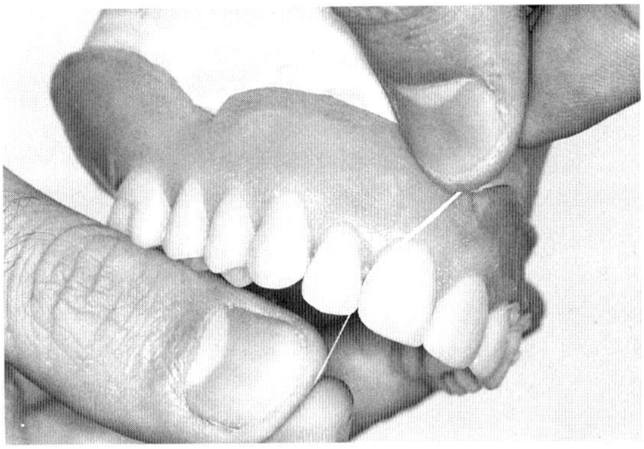

Fig. 11-12 Thin dental floss is used between the teeth to remove excess wax.

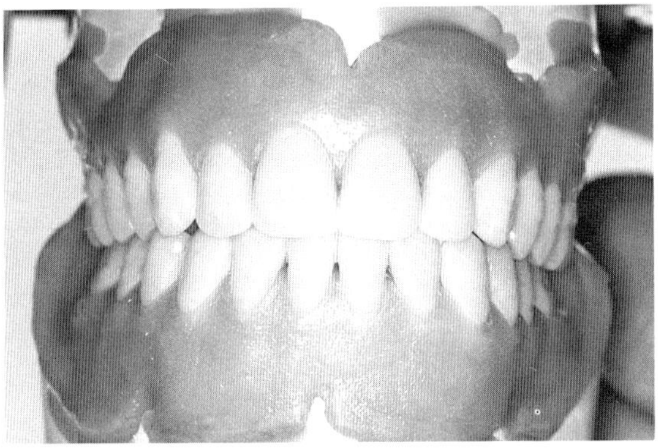

Fig. 11-13 A completed wax-up. The occlusion should be rechecked at this time.

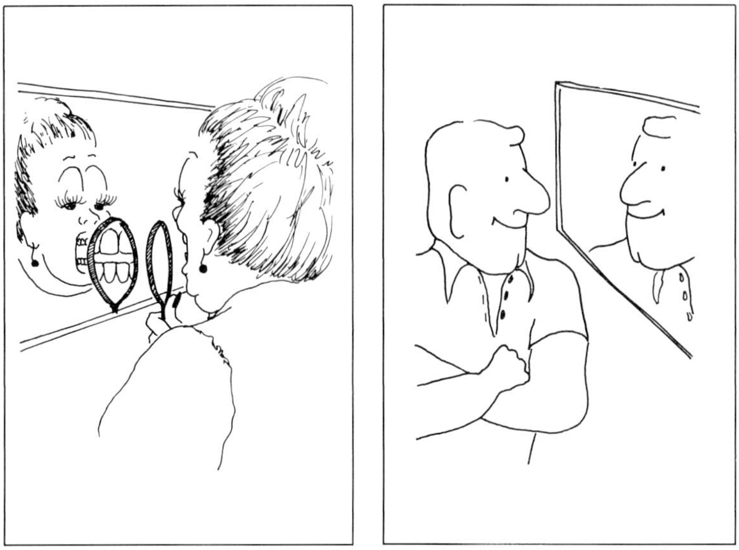

Fig. 11-14a *(left)* Some people will examine minute details of tooth arrangements.

Fig. 11-14b *(right)* Other people will not even look at their new dentures.

shrinkage could leave a space between the new and old resin. The added wax will help prevent a visible line of division between the acrylic resin being processed to the completed base.

7. Customize the maxillary palatal rugae on the completed maxillary base by visually duplicating the rugae seen on the preliminary diagnostic cast or by using alginate to duplicate the patient's rugae as found inside the completed base. If the patient prefers to have a smooth palate, this step can be eliminated, but be sure to add wax anyway to ensure proper palatal thickness. The rugae can always be removed from the completed base after processing if the patient objects to their presence. See the completed wax-up in Fig. 11-13.

The final esthetic check

Tooth selection and arrangement are now examined. The patient is not asked to inspect the dentures until they meet the dentist's approval. The following are evaluated:

1. Tooth size, mold, and color
2. Tooth arrangement (including overlaps, diastemata, and so on)
3. Individual characterization of the teeth (notches, grooves, wear, fillings, and so on)
4. Amount of tooth exposed during rest, speech, and smiling
5. Gingival contour

As mentioned in chapter 9, the objective is to make the dentures look so real that they defy detection by others as "false" teeth.

Patient approval

It is now time to have the patient, his family, and his friends look at the denture. Do not rush this time! Let the patient look at his teeth while he is standing in front of a large wall mirror rather than holding a small hand mirror. Using a large wall mirror enables the patient to see his whole face rather than just part of it. The patient will see the dentures as they relate to his whole face and upper body.

There are two opposite ways patients may look at their dentures (with many variations in between). One type of patient may run right up to the mirror, evaluate his lips, and look right at his individual teeth, while another type will approach the mirror with extreme caution and, in fact, not even look at his teeth (Figs. 11-14a and b).

The first type of patient is probably very exacting and analytical. You should encourage this type of patient to stand back a bit from the mirror to look at himself the way others will see him. That is why you should not hand this patient a small mirror. The second patient is more likely a very accommodating patient, but you must still beware. Encourage this patient to look more closely at his teeth before he accepts them. It would not be unusual for this type of patient to accept the dentures as they are set up but later find the dentures unesthetic for some reason (perhaps a friend's or relative's opinion). It is advisable to have both types of patients take home the wax-up of the trial denture so that they (with family and friends) can inspect the dentures in the privacy of their homes. Advise the patient both orally and in writing not to eat or drink anything with these teeth and to place them in for only short (10 to 15 minutes) periods for inspection. Instruct the patient to make a written list of any changes or suggestions that he may have. This step may have to be repeated several times for some patients. Now is the time to make any changes, because the teeth are easily moved in the wax.

After patient acceptance and satisfaction, you can proceed to complete the dentures. When the try-in visits are completed, the dentist can feel rewarded knowing that he has done something artistic for the patient, while the patient can feel that he has actively participated in the fabrication of his dentures. The patient must assume the responsibility for either accepting or rejecting the esthetics of the denture at this time. Completed denture bases enable the dentist to present the patient with the same esthetics the day of insertion.

References

1. Pound, E. Utilizing speech to simplify a personalized denture service. J. Prosthet. Dent. 24:586, 1970.
2. Blumenthal, E. Personal communication, 1971.
3. Academy of Denture Prosthetics. Glossary of Prosthodontic Terms. 4th ed. St. Louis: C.V. Mosby Co., 1977.

When I was in dental school, we didn't get any credit for talking to or listening to the patient. We only got credit for doing something technical to the patient. So many dentists figure that they're not doing anything unless they are making something for the patient. Now this is not true. Physicians are not trained in this way. They are supposed to talk to and listen to the patient. They realize that the less they do to the patient, perhaps the better off the patient will be. If a patient comes in and says to the physician, "I'm too fat," the physician could say, "Lie down and we'll cut off the fat and that will solve your problem." No, the physician suggests that the patient change his diet, exercise, etc. If the patient doesn't do as the physician suggests, he will simply say that the patient didn't follow his suggestions.

We as dentists don't want to impose our esthetic values upon the patient. Give the patient ample time to examine the trial dentures with the teeth set up in wax. Because the patient cannot see himself as others will see him, it is important to seek the participation of the patient's family members or friends at this time. Regardless, this is a most appropriate time to talk to and especially listen to the patient.

Allen Brewer
(Personal communication)

Chapter 12

The Second Processing

A second processing is now performed to attach the denture teeth and added wax to the completed denture base. This procedure involves first flasking the denture and then packing and processing the acrylic resin.

Brewer has shown that this second processing, when done at a reduced temperature (138°F) over an extended time period (12 hours) will result in very little dimensional change to the completed base.[1] He also has demonstrated that the greatest dimensional change of the acrylic resin takes place when the completed base is first processed, before any jaw relation records are made. Through the combined use of completed bases, accurate mounting casts, checkpoints, and the articulator remount after the second processing, the denture occlusion can be refined on the articulator so that there is no need to remount the dentures at the time of insertion.

Flasking the denture

1. Warm a piece of baseplate wax, and place the borders of the mandibular denture against the warmed wax. Using a sharp blade, follow the outline form of the denture to cut out a piece of wax to fill in the tongue space, and attach the cut wax to the mandibular base with melted baseplate wax.

2. Attach a strip of beading wax around the entire periphery of the denture just at the butt joint region.

3. Mix dental stone (or stone and slurry to accelerate the set) and pour the stone into the completed bases to make new casts within them. Invert the denture base over a base of stone to complete the cast. No separating medium is needed inside of the completed bases because the stone will not stick to the already processed acrylic resin.

4. Remove the beading wax and use a model trimmer and knives to adjust the cast. Try the cast inside of the flask to see if it fits. The land area of the cast should be smooth and at a level slightly below that of the wax. Place a thin layer of petroleum jelly on all stone surfaces.

5. Mix more stone, place it in the lower half of the flask, and insert the cast into the flask. As the stone rises around the land area of the cast, position the stone up to the land area. As the stone begins to set, remove excess stone with a lab knife and use your fingers to smooth the stone to eliminate any undercuts (Fig. 12-1). The maxillary denture base is treated slightly differently. Adapt some stone onto the posterior palatal portion of the denture (Fig. 12-2). This added stone will help secure the maxillary base on the cast so that it will not lift off during packing of the acrylic resin. This step is particularly important if there are not any undercuts on the tissue surface of the maxillary denture base.

6. Add fluid baseplate wax to any areas of the stone that are undercut to the anticipated path of withdrawal of the flasks. As a separating medium for the stone, to help minimize the thickness of

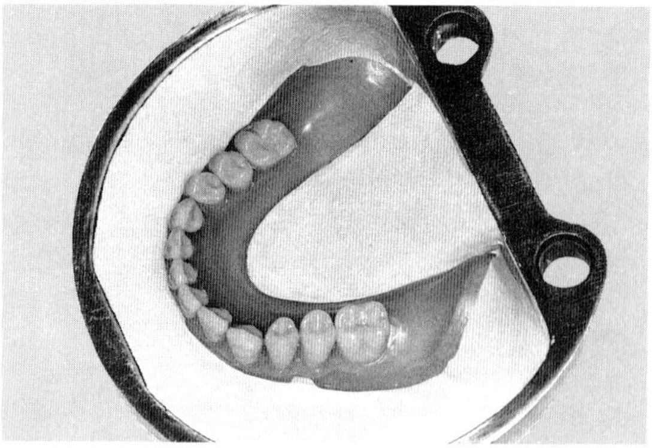

Fig. 12-1 The stone is adapted to be level with the land areas.

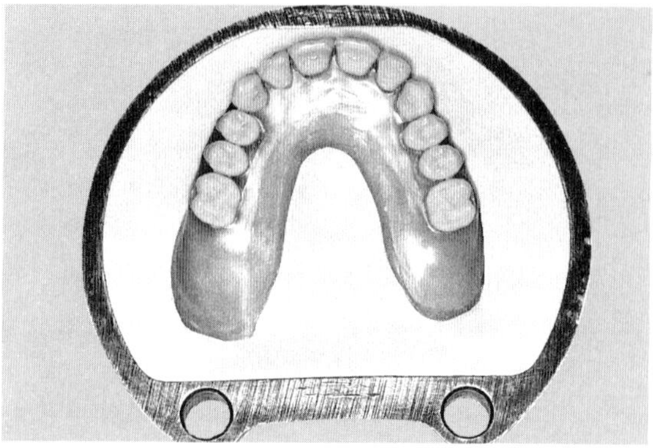

Fig. 12-2 Some stone is adapted onto the posterior palatal portion of the maxillary denture base to ensure that the base will be secure on the cast during flasking and packing.

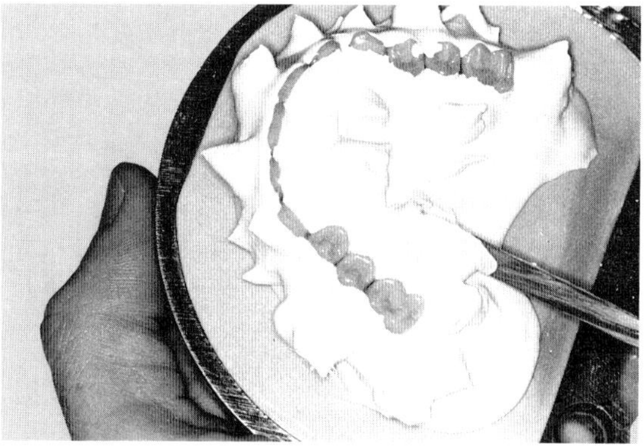

Fig. 12-3 Adapt a thin mix of stone around and between the teeth to cover the buccal and lingual surfaces of the teeth and the wax surfaces.

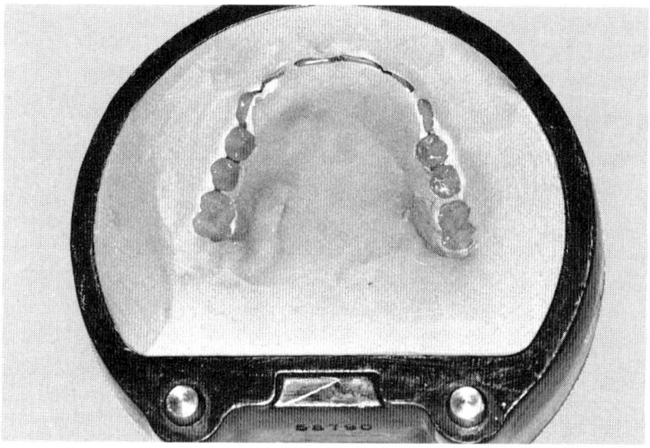

Fig. 12-4 The incisal and occlusal surfaces of the teeth are wiped clean of stone before the stone has set.

the separating layer, a 50% diluted soap solution* can be used.

7. Paint a surface tension–reducing liquid† on the wax surface of the denture. This will allow the stone to flow over the wax more efficiently and will produce fewer voids. Make a third (slightly thinner) mix of stone and use a cement spatula to adapt it around and between the teeth (Fig. 12-3). This will provide a thin (approximately one quarter inch) matrix of stone to secure the teeth while minimizing the change caused by the setting expansion of the stone as well as the heat produced by the setting stone. Wipe the stone from incisal and occlusal surfaces of the teeth before it has set (Fig. 12-4). This will enable the person deflasking to locate the teeth visually.

8. Place the top half of the flask into position, and momentarily fill the flask with water. Make a fourth mix of stone and vibrate it into the flask up to the incisal and occlusal surfaces of the teeth.

9. Place a separating solution on the stone sur-

* Ivory Liquid, Procter & Gamble, Cincinnati, Ohio.
† Perf-Cast, Buffalo Dental Mfg. Co., Brooklyn, N.Y.

faces, and pour the last mix of stone into the flask. The inside of the cover of the flask has stone adapted to it and is then placed upon the flask and closed into contact. Wipe the excess material from around the periphery of the flask and allow the stone to set.

Each mix of stone used in the flasking procedure should be an alternate color (yellow to white to yellow, for example). This will make it easier to identify each flasking stone step during the deflasking procedure. If stone and slurry are used to flask a denture, the entire denture can be flasked in one hour—each stone layer takes approximately ten minutes to set.

10. Completely immerse the flask in a pan of boiling water for five minutes. Then remove the flask and carefully pry it apart.

The wax should be soft enough at the five-minute time interval. If the denture is left too long in the hot water, the wax will be quite fluid. The wax can be lifted or peeled away and discarded rather than washed down the drain.

11. Pour clean boiling water over both halves of the flask. Use teapots filled with boiling water rather than a "boil-out tank." It is easy for boil-out tanks to become contaminated with wax residue. Use a pastry brush to clean all stone surfaces with a liquid soap solution. Repeat this procedure involving boiling water and liquid soap two or more times to ensure that the stone surfaces and denture teeth are clean and free of all contaminants. If a wax film remains on the surface of the acrylic resin teeth, there will not be an effective chemical bond of the teeth to the acrylic resin.

12. Roughen the undersurface of acrylic resin denture teeth (if acrylic resin teeth were used) to eliminate the shiny, uncut surface. In addition, use a No. 2 round bur to place several small holes on the ridge lap areas of the teeth. The small holes will provide additional bonding area for the acrylic resin. The roughened surface will significantly enhance the bond strength between the acrylic resin teeth and the acrylic resin of the denture base.

13. Check the completed denture base in the other half of the flask to determine if the butt joint is present around the entire base and to verify that all contaminants have been removed.

14. Paint one layer of tinfoil substitute* on all stone surfaces. Be careful not to let any tinfoil substitute get on the ridge lap areas of the acrylic resin teeth. This can also significantly affect the bond strength between the acrylic resins. Although some suggest that a second layer of tinfoil substitute be applied after the first layer has dried,[2] we have found this to be unnecessary.

15. Mix the shade of heat-curing acrylic resin that matches the shade of the acrylic resin used for the completed base (30 cc of powder to 12 ml of liquid for the average maxillary or mandibular denture—check the manufacturer's directions for exact proportions). Should any gingival toning be desired, do it at this time.

Using a small brush, wet the acrylic resin teeth with monomer immediately prior to placing the acrylic resin in the flask. When the acrylic resin reaches the doughy stage, manually adapt it into the half of the flask containing the denture teeth. Place one large sheet of cellophane (6 inch by 6 inch Densilk 1-m sheets†) over one half of the flask, and place the other half of the flask over it with some manual pressure. Then place the flask in the bench press and *slowly* close it. This is important because too fast a closure can result in tooth movement caused by too much pressure.

Once you have closed the flask as far as it will go with moderate pressure (usually over one to two minutes), release the bench press and open the flask. An excess of acrylic resin material (often called the "flash") should be found around the entire land area. If excess is not seen everywhere, the flask is likely underpacked. If this is the case, add additional acrylic resin before the next closure of the flask.

The excess of flash should be removed with a sharp blade so that the flask can be completely closed. Additional excess acrylic resin will keep the two halves of the flask from having metal-to-metal contact, thus increasing the chances of altering the pin opening after the dentures are processed. Should the acrylic resin appear too thin in any

*Al-cote, L.D. Caulk Co., Milford, Del.
†Reliance Dental Mfg. Co., Worth, Ill.

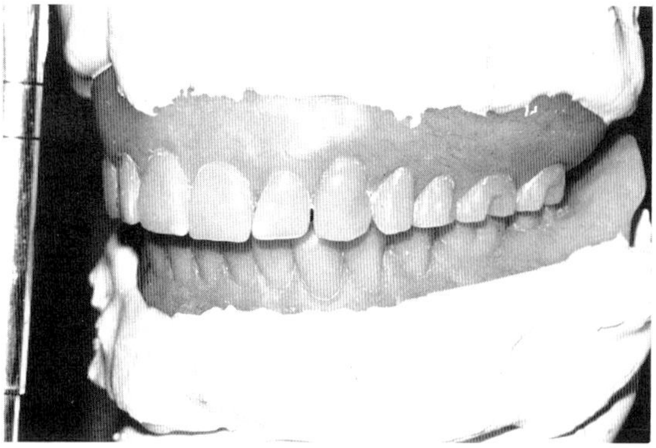

Fig. 12-5 The dentures are secured to the mounting casts with sticky wax and then with stone and slurry.

areas where resin is needed, the corresponding area on the completed denture bases should be reduced using a carbide bur. This will ensure that a bulk of acrylic resin will be added for good bonding and an esthetic result.

Place another single sheet of cellophane between the two halves of the flask and again close it and place it in the bench press. This time, apply more pressure because there is much less resistance from excess acrylic resin.

16. Remove the flask from the bench press again and repeat step 15. It may take, on the average, three to four closures before the flask is completely closed.

17. Paint the completed denture base half of the flask with monomer immediately before the final closure of the flask. Once this is done, close the flasks together (with *no* cellophane strips) and then replace them in the bench press and close them under heavy pressure.

18. Place the flasks in a curing compress and allow them to bench cure for 15 minutes before placing them in a cold-curing tank. Close the flask compress completely using the supplied wrench and then open it approximately a one-quarter turn so that the spring can be activated to allow for expansion of the flask and its contents. Process the acrylic resin for a minimum of 12 hours at 138°F. If more time is available, cure the acrylic resin for up to 20 to 24 hours. Following processing, remove the denture compress from the curing tank and allow it to bench cool to room temperature before deflasking.

19. Deflask the denture in the conventional manner. When all the stone has been removed, place the dentures in an ultrasonic bath containing stone and plaster remover solution for ten to 15 minutes.

20. Remove any excess flash from the dentures. Then place the dentures back on the mounting casts. Be sure that no debris (wax or stone) is on the periphery of the mounting casts. Secure the dentures to the remount casts by using first sticky wax and then stone and slurry (Fig. 12-5). The dentures should not move from the mounting casts during the grind-in process.

21. Close the articulator until the first tooth contact is made, and then note the position of the incisal guide pin in relation to the guide table (see Fig. 10-1). Using articulating paper, mark the occlusal interferences in the centric position and adjust the occlusion in this position until the incisal guide pin touches the incisal guide table. It should be remembered that when adjusting the occlusion in the centric jaw relation position, the centric holding cusps (buccal of the mandible and the lingual of the maxilla) are not altered. The lateral excursions are refined using the rule of *BULL* (Buccal of the Uppers; Lingual of the Lowers) on the working side; therefore, adjust the buccal cusps of the maxilla and the lingual cusps of the mandible. Adjust all nonworking interferences. Make protrusive movements and appropriately adjust the occlusion. The amount and nature of occlusal refinement depends upon the philosophy and technique of occlusion used.

22. Apply milling and polishing cream (Justi Milling and Polishing Creme*) for acrylic resin teeth or carborundum paste (Rapid Cutting Abrasive Paste†) for porcelain teeth to the occlusal and incisal surfaces of the teeth. Then move the articulator approximately five times to each side in the working motion, followed by the protrusive position. Repeat until smooth, gliding movements can be made. Do not use the paste until the teeth have

*H.D. Justi Co., Oxnard, Calif.
†Kerr Dental Mfg. Co., Romulus, Mich.

already been appropriately ground-in using a grinding stone.

23. Complete the remount procedure by rechecking the occlusion in the centric position. Place the thin (13-μm) Artus* strips between all the teeth on both sides to make sure that there is even, firm tooth contact.

24. Remove the dentures from the mounting casts, and finish and polish them. Smooth the region of the butt joint with an acrylic resin carbide finishing bur. Remove the excess of acrylic resin that extends past the butt joint so that no thin flash is evident. With proper attention to detail, this junction of acrylic resin at the butt joint should be practically imperceptible. Polish the teeth to achieve appropriate smoothness without altering the occlusion.

25. Stipple the labial and buccal surfaces of the dentures, if desired, with bent No. 4 and No. 8 round burs. Bend the burs by placing the ends of the burs under a Bunsen burner until red hot and then bending them with a pliers to the angle desired. The burs are then used in a handpiece or a lathe and rotated in a circular motion against the acrylic resin surface. Use the smaller bur for papilla areas between the teeth and the larger bur for the remainder of the acrylic resin. Stippling in this manner creates a natural appearance of the denture surfaces because it decreases the amount of light reflection off them should the patient have a high smile line and show gingiva.

The dentures are now ready for patient insertion. They should be stored in water until the patient visit. Be sure to save the mounting casts until after the dentures have been delivered.

*Artus Co., Englewood, N.J.

References

1. Brewer, A.A. Prosthodontic research in progress at the School of Aerospace Medicine. J. Prosthet. Dent. 13:49, 1963.
2. Boucher, C.O. (ed.) Swenson's Complete Dentures. 6th ed. St. Louis: C.V. Mosby Co., 1970.

There are two ways to fabricate complete dentures—before insertion and after insertion. We want the dentures to be correct before insertion.

Allen Brewer
(Personal communication)

Chapter 13

Denture Insertion and Maintenance

The insertion appointment takes only a few minutes. Efforts invested in the earlier phases now provide the reward of a relaxing and effective insertion visit. Factors such as stability, retention, fit, and comfort of the denture bases have already been examined via the completed bases. The vertical dimension, centric jaw relation/centric occlusion, occlusal scheme, esthetics, and phonetics have been verified as correct in advance of the insertion visit. This visit should be a pleasant, essentially nonworking session for both the dentist and the patient. The patient can be given final oral and written instructions regarding wearing and caring for complete dentures. Whenever possible, schedule the patient for a 24-hour recall.

Postinsertion maintenance

Postinsertion maintenance care of a denture patient is as important for the patient as are the procedures used to fabricate the dentures. Maintenance after denture insertion can often be the key to denture success. The patient *must have scheduled appointments* for his recall visits.

During the diagnosis and treatment planning visits, the patient should be advised that his dentures will require maintenance and *scheduled postinsertion* visits. It should not be a surprise to the patient when on the day of insertion you ask him to return the next day or a following day for a postinsertion visit. The patient should be advised of the need for and benefits of these additional visits. If this need is communicated clearly to the patient during the first diagnostic visit and reinforced during the remaining treatment, the patient will be more adequately prepared psychologically to return for regularly scheduled recall visits and not be surprised if some discomfort is encountered.

Scheduling of postinsertion visits

A routine appointment should be made for examination and adjustment *within 24 hours* of denture insertion. This is a *critical period* for a denture patient. Careful attention at this time will often minimize postinsertion problems and provide encouragement to the patient. Sensitive areas of irritation can often be identified at this time and adjusted before the patient experiences discomfort and mental anguish or anger. Other than scheduled appointments, ask the patient to call for an appointment if any problems arise in the interim.

If during the first appointment no adjustments or only minor corrections are required, the patient should be given another appointment for a week later. It is difficult to establish a recall schedule for patients in general; rather, recalls should be tailored to each patient. However, if pronounced tissue irritation is seen at the first adjustment period, adjustments should be made and the patient given an appointment for the following day or two. The patient should be given definite adjustment appointments as required, until such time as patient comfort is ensured and the dentures no longer appear to be a source of tissue irritation.

Equipment and supplies

You should have the following equipment and supplies available for postinsertion visits:

1. Articulating paper
2. Dr. Thompson's Color Transfer Applicators*
3. Pressure-indicating paste with brush applicator
4. Pear-, egg-, and flame-shaped acrylic carbide laboratory burs
5. No. 4 and No. 8 round burs
6. No. 557 fissure bur

Pressure-indicating paste can also be made by combining two cups of Crisco† with two cups of zinc oxide powder.[2]

Clinical procedures

Ask the patient to describe his experiences with his new dentures. Listen carefully. The patient's comments may provide help in evaluating speech, functional, or psychological problems.

If the patient has had a problem, ask him to describe it. If there are several problems, write them down while the patient describes them. This not only avoids the possibility of forgetting to correct one of them, but also shows the patient you are truly concerned.

Be careful about removing the dentures from the patient's mouth. The patient is usually more adept at avoiding sensitive areas when removing the dentures, so let him remove the dentures and place them on the bracket table without handing them to you. Rinse clean the dentures and return them to the bracket table.

Perform a careful intraoral exam of the tissues. Dry the tissues with 2 inch × 2 inch gauze for this inspection. Meticulously examine the tissues. You can also instruct the patient to point to areas that are bothering him.

The most frequent causes of irritation are pressure areas within the denture, overextensions of the periphery, and failure to provide relief for nonyielding areas or areas overlying nerves and blood vessels, such as greater palatine and nasopalatine foramina. Reddened areas are usually the result of an acute irritation. White areas are usually the result of chronic irritation.

*Great Plains Dental Products Co., Kingman, Kan.
†Proctor & Gamble, Cincinnati, Ohio.

Procedure to use if you can see the sore area

Dry tissue in the area of the sore spot with 2 inch × 2 inch gauze. Use a Thompson marking stick to mark precisely the sore area. (You can wet the top of the marker on a piece of wet gauze.)

Insert the *dried denture* in the mouth to transfer the marking to the denture. If the denture is wet, the mark usually smudges to a large, broad area away from the sore. Remove, examine, and evaluate the denture. Use appropriate burs to relieve the area to which the ink was transferred.

Procedure to use with pressure-indicating paste

Pressure-indicating paste (PIP*) can also be used to determine whether the area of discomfort is being caused by excessive pressure of an area of the denture. Overextensions of the denture borders can also be evaluated with PIP. Place PIP on the denture in the area of the soreness or overextension. Place the denture in the mouth. Ask the patient to close his teeth together and to swallow some water. You can also activate an area, as in border molding, to help determine if there is an overextension. Allow the denture to be in place for several minutes with the indicating paste if the area is difficult to locate.

Repolishing the adjusted areas

Repolish the areas that were ground on the outer polished surface of the denture. The areas that were adjusted on the inner impressioned tissue surface of the denture should be polished with a soft rubber wheel. Reinsert the dentures and ask the patient how he feels. The patient may still feel uncomfortable because the area remains irritated from

*Mizzy Co., Clifton Forge, Va.

previous soreness. Usually there is some sense of relief if the problem area was correctly identified.

Many problems may arise during the postinsertion appointment. During this time, differential diagnosis must be made to help determine the cause of the patient's discomfort or dissatisfaction. Prior to dismissing the patient, ask if he has any questions or concerns. It is wise to again reinforce the home care instructions that you gave your patient the day before.

The patient should be scheduled for a recall examination approximately 6 to 12 months later if there are no further problems. The patient should be encouraged to call if he has any problems prior to that time.

To conclude, the patient must understand that the preservation of remaining oral tissues is just as important for the edentulous patient as it is for the patient with natural teeth. Periodic recall examinations enable the dentist to evaluate his procedures as well as incorporate important preventive concepts into his practice.

Denture maintenance

It is important at the time of insertion that a patient be thoroughly informed about the care of his prosthesis. Inadequately cleaned dentures can result in tissue irritation and stained teeth and denture bases, with resulting odors.

Dentures may be kept relatively clean by using a soft-bristled brush and soap and water after each meal and before bedtime. Other denture paste cleaners and regular dentifrice act primarily by an abrasive action. Care should be taken that they are not too abrasive. Because cleaning after each meal may be impractical for working people, rinsing under tap water may be all that is possible. Deposits accumulate at varying rates depending upon each patient's habits and the physiology of the oral environment. Therefore, more complex procedures than simple brushing may be necessary. Others may prefer to use some type of immersion solutions.

Commercial solutions may be useful for the removal of superficial debris and for daily use with new dentures. However, for heavier accumulations, other methods may be required. Some solutions contain a hypochlorite ingredient that is very effective in removing plaque; however, it should not be used with soft liners, metal bases, or frameworks used with removable partial dentures. Carbon dioxide–producing bicarbonate cleaners (such as Polident* and Efferdent†) are easy to use and not harmful to soft liners and metal frameworks, but may not be as effective in plaque removal. If using any type of commercial solution, the patient should follow the manufacturer's instructions and then brush the prosthesis after its removal from the solution. This will remove any loose debris as well as any traces of the cleaning solution. Some patients' tissues may be sensitive to the bicarbonates or hypochlorites found in the cleaners.

Home cleansing agents can be used if prepared properly. A solution of one part Chlorox,‡ two parts Calgon,¶ and eight parts water can be very effective in removing plaque.[1] It should not be used with soft liners or metal frameworks because of sodium hypochlorite in the Chlorox. Tenacious deposits that are not removed by conventional commercial methods should be removed by professional ultrasonic cleaning devices. To date, home sonic cleaners are not that beneficial. It appears that their effectiveness is related to their chemical activity, not their vibrating action.

No matter how the denture is cleaned, when it is not in the mouth for extended periods of time it should be kept in a moist environment. Room-temperature tap water is all that is necessary.

In addition to care of the prosthesis, the patient should be informed about the care of the soft tissue. The dentures should not be worn both night and day. For many patients, leaving the dentures out at night allows the tissues to be stimulated by the tongue and saliva. For others, leaving the dentures out during daytime may be more convenient. Leaving the dentures out for four to six hours can allow for a healthier mucosa. Patients that cannot or will not leave the dentures out for extended time periods should be instructed in massaging the denture-bearing areas with a soft-bristled brush.

*Block Drug Co., Jersey City, N.J.
†Warner Lambert Co., Morris Plains, N.J.
‡The Chlorox Co., Oakland, Calif.
¶Beecham Products, Pittsburgh, Pa.

References

1. Ghalichebaf, M., Graser, G.N., and Zander, H.A. The efficacy of denture cleansing agents. J. Prosthet. Dent. 48:515–520, 1982.
2. Gronas, D.G. Preparation of pressure indicating paste. J. Prosthet. Dent. 37:92, 1977.

The patient may be reevaluated in a week, a month, six months, a year, or two years. At least we want the patient to know that his treatment is never completed. I am horrified to see some of the dentures I made ten years ago. The patient changes, society changes, we change and only by constant reevaluation of all factors can we hope to provide optimum denture service.

Allen Brewer
(From: Selection of denture teeth for esthetics and function. J. Prosthet. Dent. 23:373, 1970.)

Chapter 14

Removable Partial Dentures

Making removable partial dentures can be a very rewarding experience, but at the same time it can be extremely frustrating. There are so many clinical and laboratory technical procedures that can go wrong. Compared to making a removable partial denture, getting a single cast crown to fit one tooth could be considered simple (Fig. 14-1).

In fabricating a removable partial denture, 16 essential clinical and/or laboratory steps are accomplished by the dentist and the laboratory technician (Table 14-1). Each of the 16 steps is important, and the responsibilities for the completed removable partial denture are divided quite evenly between the dentist and the laboratory technician. The success of each step is dependent upon the steps that precede it. Therefore, a good working relationship and clear communication between the dentist and the laboratory technician are necessary.

The material presented here on removable partial dentures is not meant to be a comprehensive treatise on removable partial dentures, because other publications cover the core material quite adequately. Rather, this section will highlight the most significant problem areas that are encountered while making removable partial dentures and will detail how completed denture bases and checkpoints are used with removable partial dentures.

Diagnostic casts

The importance of accurate and neat diagnostic casts is stressed in all dental education. This emphasis is particularly justified when a removable partial denture is being planned. In addition, it is sometimes necessary to mount the diagnostic casts on an articulator to get a better view of the interarch occlusal relationships.

We look for several things on mounted diagnostic casts. *Supererupted teeth* in the opposing arch can complicate the fabrication of a removable partial denture. These supererupted teeth may leave inadequate room to place the framework, the acrylic resin base material, or the denture teeth (Fig. 14-2). Tooth cusps may contact the opposing teeth exactly in the position where an occlusal, incisal, or cingulum rest is being considered. The rest seat preparations should be made by reducing enough tooth structure, or the opposing dentition should be reduced. It is sometimes necessary to place the rest on a different tooth surface. When a removable partial denture is completed and inserted, the partial denture framework or the attached teeth must not keep the other natural or denture teeth from contacting in appropriate occlusion (Fig. 14-3).

The rest seats must be properly located so that the occlusion is not changed when the removable partial denture is inserted. During the framework try-in (with no teeth yet attached to the framework), check first to see the location and intensity of tooth contacts when the removable partial denture is out of the mouth. Use mylar tape strips (13 μm thick) cut into 2-mm-wide pieces. Instruct the patient to close onto this tape, and then pull up on it to see whether the opposing teeth are in contact. Then

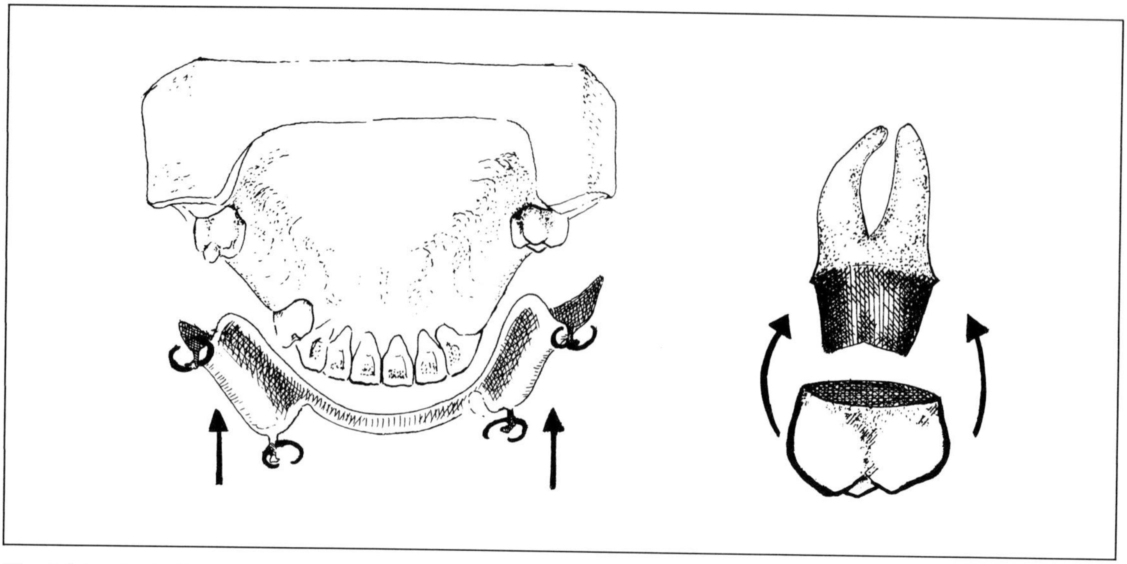

Fig. 14-1 A single cast crown *(left)* has to fit only one tooth, whereas a removable partial denture casting *(right)* must contact multiple teeth accurately.

Table 14-1 The 16 essential clinical and laboratory steps to fabricate a removable partial denture

Procedure	Accomplished by: Dentist	Accomplished by: Technician
Examination, diagnosis, and prognosis	√	
Survey and design	√	
Mouth (tooth) preparation	√	
Impressioning	√	
Master cast preparation		√
Duplication of master cast and making of refractory cast		√
Wax-up of partial denture upon refractory cast and investing		√
Casting of framework		√
Finishing and polishing of framework and fitting casting to master cast		√
Evaluating casting upon cast and teeth	√	
Altered cast impressioning	√	
Determining jaw relations	√	
Tooth setup		√
Try-in of tooth arrangement	√	
Processing of acrylic resin		√
Insertion	√	

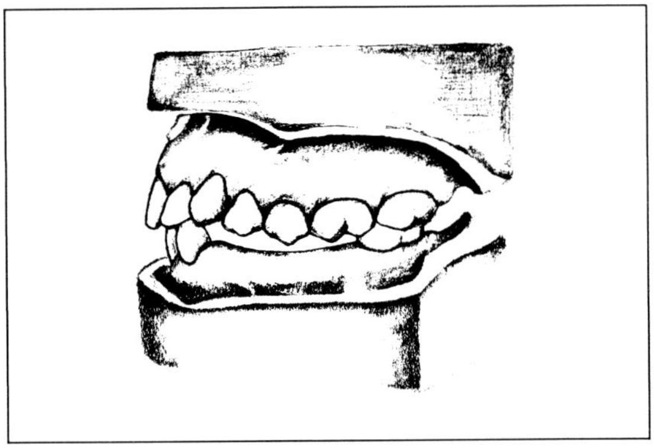

Fig. 14-2 Supererupted teeth may not leave enough room to position the framework, the acrylic resin denture base material, or the denture teeth.

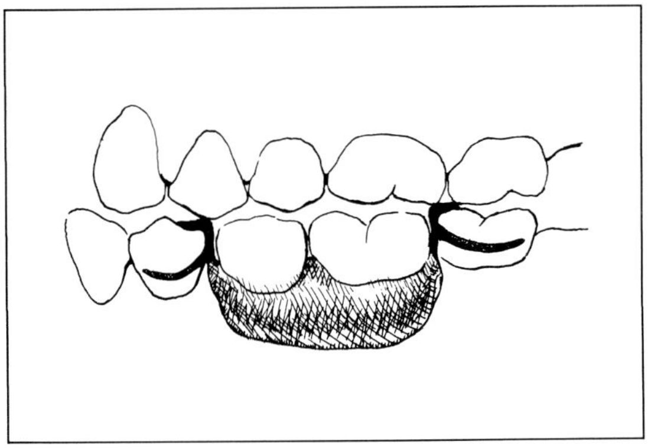

Fig. 14-3 The partial denture framework is keeping the teeth from contacting as they do when no removable partial denture is in place.

insert the framework and recheck the tooth contacts. The contacts should be the same when the removable partial denture is in the mouth. It may be necessary to adjust the opposing dentition in some areas or to grind the framework. Do not depend too much upon grinding the metal framework, because this may make the metal too thin and susceptible to fracture. The metal should be at least 1 mm thick in all areas of the occlusal rest.

Surveying

Survey the diagnostic and working casts to determine the most appropriate path of insertion for the removable partial denture. The surveyor is useful in determining if sufficient undercut exists on a tooth to provide adequate retention. The heights of contour on each tooth surface are marked with a carbon rod. The best placement of the cast on the surveyor is such that the occlusal plane is perpendicular to the vertical rod of the surveyor (Fig. 14-4). This position on the surveyor will ensure retention for the removable partial denture to the path of withdrawal if sticky foods pull upon the partial denture to dislodge it. Tilting the cast on the surveyor table may provide for retention to that path on the surveyor, but not when the partial denture is in the mouth. The cast can be tilted slightly to help equalize the depth of the undercuts on the teeth to be clasped, to improve the esthetics of the partial denture, or to minimize soft tissue interference. If appropriate undercuts are not present, the abutment teeth must be recontoured or restored. When anterior teeth are missing, the cast is usually tilted posteriorly to minimize the interference of the anterior ridge and to improve the

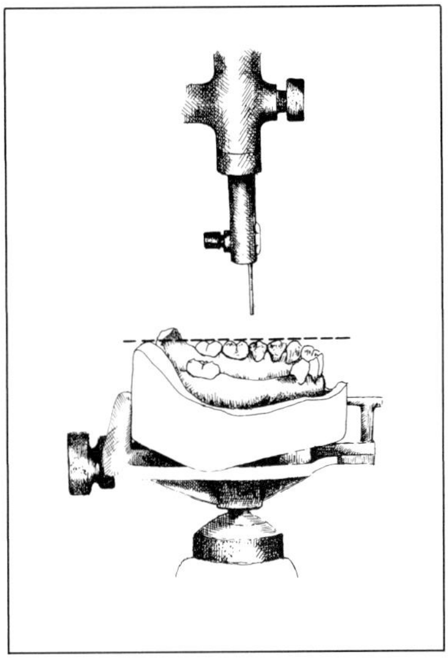

Fig. 14-4 The best position for the cast on the surveyor is such that the occlusal plane is perpendicular to the vertical rod of the surveyor. This provides retention in the path of withdrawal if sticky foods dislodge the partial denture.

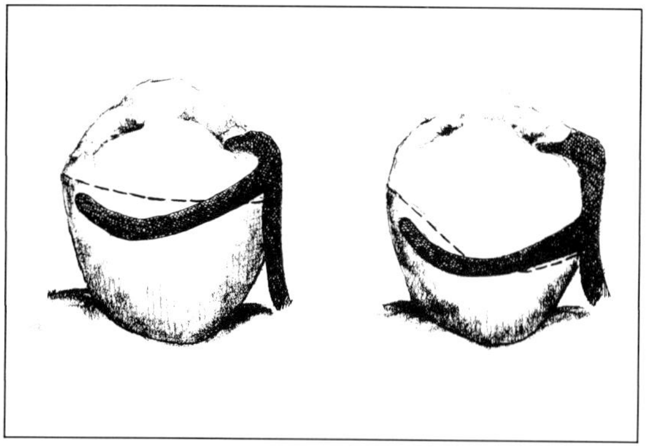

Fig. 14-5 *(left)* The clasp arm originates from the minor connector close to the occlusal rest; this is incorrect. *(right)* When a favorable height of contour exists, the clasp arm can originate from the middle portion of the minor connector.

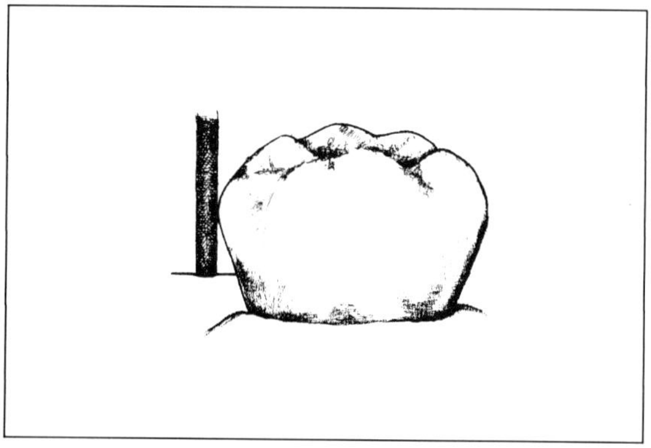

Fig. 14-6 Undercut areas to be used by flexible components of the clasps are located using undercut gauges.

appearance of the partial denture by allowing the labial flange to approximate the labial portion of the ridge. The proximal or lingual surfaces of the teeth, which will serve as guiding surfaces parallel to the path of insertion, are also considered.

The buccal and lingual heights of contour of the teeth are marked with a carbon rod. Unfavorable heights of contour would force you to position the clasps at too occlusal a level. When unfavorable heights of contour exist on the teeth, the clasp arms originate from the minor connectors quite close to the occlusal rests rather than from the middle portion of the minor connector (Fig. 14-5). When the clasp arm originates from the middle portion of the minor connector, it will be more esthetic because it will be more gingival and more likely to be out of sight when the patient speaks or smiles. Also, the forces generated by the clasp arms would be lower on the tooth and therefore closer to the center of rotation.

The areas of tooth undercut used for retention are located by using the appropriate undercut gauges (Fig. 14-6).

It is important to remember that we *cannot* make an undercut by using an exaggerated tilt of the cast on the surveyor table. The tilt of the cast should be such that the occlusal plane of the teeth is parallel to the floor. This will be the position of the teeth in the mouth relative to the path of removal when foods tend to unseat the partial denture when it is in the mouth. At this pitch and placement on the surveyor table, the located undercuts will be active only when attempting to remove the partial denture from the mouth.

A minimum tilt of the cast is also important so that the patient can insert the removable partial denture with ease and not at an awkward angle. Remember that an undercut should not be made by tilting the cast; rather, this tilting can reposition the undercut.

Intraoral surveying

Extraoral surveying of stone casts, as discussed, enables one to mark the heights of contour upon the teeth of the diagnostic casts. Intraoral surveying, as we will use the concept here, is an adjunct to, not a substitute for, extraoral surveying. Intraoral surveying is used as a guideline to duplicate what has been accomplished on the diagnostic casts. A technique for intraoral surveying will be described that enables one to mark survey lines directly on the teeth that are to be prepared. An inexpensive instrument that can be effectively used for intraoral surveying will be described.

Intraoral surveying of the abutment teeth for the removable partial denture should be accomplished prior to any tooth recontouring or preparation with burs. Intraoral surveying is approached using exactly the same rationale as is used for the extraoral surveying of stone casts.

Jermyn has described a technique by which mouth preparation for fixed partial dentures can be accomplished with the use of a precision paralleling device.[1] Using a paralleling device (Parallaid*), all of the reductions of tooth structure in an axial plane are made with the handpiece and bur locked into a paralleling device. This method of tooth reduction converts "by eye," freehand tooth reduction into a precise milling procedure.

The intraoral surveyor is by no means as precise as the Parallaid paralleling device or an extraoral surveyor. The accuracy of the intraoral surveyor can be better compared to that of a freehand, operator-manipulated bur on a handpiece. Nevertheless, the intraoral surveyor adds a guideline that would otherwise not be there.

Intraoral surveying is used to accomplish the following objectives both prior to and after completion of tooth recontouring:

1. To locate the most favorable path of intraoral insertion
2. To mark the position of the height of contour on the abutment teeth
3. To locate and measure the undercuts available for retention

The intraoral surveyor is an excellent instrument for demonstrating to students where tooth recontouring is necessary directly on the tooth to be prepared. As mentioned previously, intraoral surveying is not a substitute for extraoral surveying. Rather, it provides direction and adds control to the intraoral mouth preparation.

Alginate impressions for new diagnostic casts made after mouth (tooth) preparation has been completed are also a reliable method of rechecking the adequacy of mouth preparation on an extraoral surveyor. *If additional mouth preparation is still necessary, the intraoral surveyor can be used to mark the same areas intraorally to provide a visual guideline.*

* Jermyn Co., Rochester, N.Y.

A carbon rod can be inserted between the scissor end of blunted hemostats. Be careful not to close the hemostats too hard because the carbon rod could fracture. The carbon rod can be wrapped in paper toweling prior to closure to prevent its being fractured. Be certain to place a gauze pack behind the rod to prevent its aspiration if the carbon rod breaks. An alternative instrument can be made out of many of the contra-angle toothpick holders that are available. The hole would have to be widened to permit the carbon rod to be inserted and held with appropriate tension.

Technique

1. Position the patient's head so that the occlusal plane of the arch that you are working on is parallel to the floor when the mouth is opened to a comfortable working position.
2. Insert an analyzing rod* in the intraoral surveyor.
3. Orient the analyzing rod to determine a selected path of insertion. Use a finger rest to maintain the analyzing rod in the same plane as you reposition the rod from tooth to tooth. This is similar to using a handpiece to prepare the teeth for fixed abutments.
4. Determine the relative parallelism of the proximal tooth surfaces by contacting the appropriate tooth surfaces with the analyzing rod.
5. Change the position of the analyzing rod anteroposteriorly until the proximal surfaces are in as near a parallel position as possible against the "future" guiding planes. This determines the path of insertion of the partial denture.
6. Rotate the analyzing rod onto the buccal and lingual surfaces of the teeth using the selected path of insertion.
7. Insert the carbon marking rod* and supporting sheath* in the intraoral surveyor.
8. Position the carbon rod against the proximal tooth surfaces to reestablish the same path of insertion.
9. Rotate the carbon rod circumferentially

*J.M. Ney Co., Bloomfield, Conn.

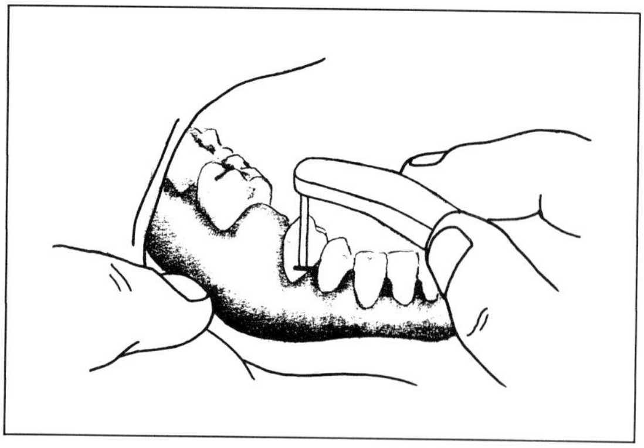

Fig. 14-7 The carbon rod is moved circumferentially around the teeth to mark the height of contour on the teeth.

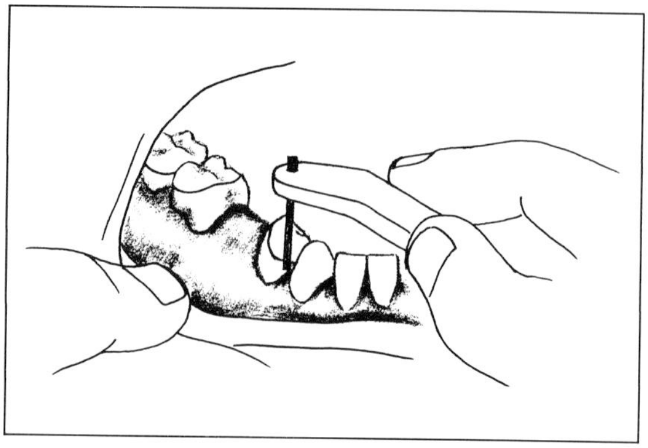

Fig. 14-8 The undercut gauges are inserted in the intraoral surveyor and the location of undercuts are determined directly on the teeth.

around the teeth to be contacted by the removable partial denture. This will mark the height of contour in pencil directly on the tooth surface (Fig. 14-7).

10. Insert the indicated undercut gauges* in the intraoral surveyor (Fig. 14-8).

11. Position the undercut gauge using the selected path of insertion. Place the undercut gauge against the tooth surface to be evaluated, and analyze the location and the amount of undercut available.

Mouth preparation using an intraoral surveyor

With the heights of contour marked directly on the tooth surfaces, it is easy to identify the intraoral areas of tooth surfaces needing recontouring. *It is an excellent visual approach for teaching purposes to identify for the student where recontouring is indicated intraorally.*

If there is an inadequate amount of undercut available on the existing tooth for a retentive clasp, the area needing recontouring is easily located. The guesswork of where to recontour is eliminated. After the tooth is recontoured with a bur, it can be rechecked for proper contour with the intraoral surveyor.

To illustrate the use of the intraoral surveyor, examples of commonly seen clinical problems and their solutions using the intraoral surveyor will be highlighted.

Problem: The height of contour of the tooth is located too high occlusally. As mentioned, in this situation the rigid and semirigid portions of the clasp (the nonflexing portions) would be too occlusal. This can result in unfavorable forces being distributed to the tooth and can lead to occlusal interferences with the opposing arch. A clasp that is too occlusal can also be unesthetic.

Solution: Mark the height of contour on the abutment tooth with the intraoral surveyor. Prepare or recontour the tooth using this line as a guide to lower the survey line for a more favorable height of contour for clasping.

Problem: An undercut exists on the tooth, but it is not adequate for retention.

Solution: Mark the height of contour on the abutment tooth with the intraoral surveyor. Place the appropriate undercut gauge on the intraoral surveyor, and insert it against the tooth. Locate and mark the area that needs recontouring to intensify the amount of undercut. Recontour the tooth and then recheck it to verify that the proper undercut has been achieved.

Problem: No undercut exists on an abutment

*J.M. Ney Co., Bloomfield, Conn.

tooth where a retentive clasp must be used. A full crown to achieve an undercut has been contraindicated.

Solution: Mark the height of contour on the abutment tooth with the intraoral surveyor. Locate and mark the area that needs recontouring. The tooth can either be recontoured to acheive an appropriate undercut or grooved or "dimpled." Prepare the tooth with recontouring or dimpling and then recheck the tooth with the appropriate undercut gauge.

These procedures enable one to scribe survey lines directly on the teeth to be used as abutments for a removable partial denture. Appropriate undercuts can also be determined by using undercut gauges directly on the tooth.

Design

A design clearly drawn on a surveyed diagnostic cast is perhaps the best way to communicate your design of the removable partial denture to the laboratory technician. This designed diagnostic cast can be sent to the dental laboratory along with the master cast and laboratory prescription. A laboratory prescription (work authorization) is a written direction for laboratory procedures to be performed in the fabrication of dental restoration.

Clearly written and detailed laboratory prescriptions are an important factor in the success of the working relationship between the dentist and the laboratory technician and in the quality of the work that is done. It is not uncommon for lack of communication to result in repeated disputes and unsatisfactory work.

Writing complete and descriptive laboratory prescriptions is both time-consuming and laborious for the dentist. The dentist is often so rushed during a busy day that information is lacking in the prescription. When details are missing in the prescription, the laboratory technician does not have enough information to do the work. The technician must either make decisions by himself to finish the work or ask the dentist for additional instructions. Often dentists write very long, detailed instructions in paragraph form. From the laboratory technician's point of view, reading lengthy prescriptions is time-consuming and confusing. The technician may not have the patience to read all the details, and often important information is hidden within a paragraph of the prescription.

A checklist laboratory form for prescription writing is an easy way to communicate. Such forms leave adequate room for any additional details that are necessary. The dentist is not burdened by writing "please" and "thank you" on each prescription. Also, the name, address, and license number of the dentist are on each form (Fig. 14-9).

Design considerations

Because so many different design concepts for removable partial dentures appear to be clinically successful, it is apparent that there is no one best type of major connector, clasp, clasp position, rest, or rest position. However, there are some critical factors in the design of a removable partial denture that, if not taken into consideration, can lead to significant problems. The design must take into consideration the health of the supporting structures—tooth and ridge areas, patient comfort, and esthetics.

There must be rigid major and minor connectors. These connectors must have adequate thickness so that they do not flex when the patient functions with the partial denture. Rigid connectors permit forces to be distributed throughout the arch (to both the teeth and tissue), avoiding undue stress concentration in any one area. The greater the length of the distal extension bases, the more bulk of metal needed to provide adequate rigidity. For patient comfort it is better to have the palatal or lingual bar connectors wide and thin rather than narrow and thick. The thicker areas may feel bulky to the patient's tongue.

The location of the mandibular and maxillary major connectors is another critical factor. The superior edge of the mandibular lingual bar should be kept approximately 3 mm away from the free gingival margin (Fig. 14-10). This distance from the free gingival margin places the bar at a lower level and at a distance where it may be less per-

FROM: Dr. John Doe (MA License No. AXG89)
4414 Mockingbird Lane
Bristol, MA 02115
Telephone: (617) XXX-XXXX

TO: X and Y Dental Lab
98 Silver Street
Freeport, MA 02115
Telephone: (617) XXX-XXXX

Date: ________________

Patient's name (or Identification no.) ________________ Age ______ Sex ______

Date and time work wanted by ________________

PRESCRIPTION

___ Call me before beginning work
___ Pour impression
___ Cast chrome framework:
 Maxillary
 Mandibular
___ Transitional RPD
___ Major connector type ________
___ All–acrylic resin partial
___ Precision; semiprecision framework
___ Designed diagnostic cast enclosed
___ Master cast surveyed and tripoded
___ Acrylic resin base(s) for:
 Impressions
 Jaw relation records
___ Altered cast
___ Tooth setup
___ Final wax-up
___ Denture base acrylic resin to use ________
___ Processing
___ Finish and polish
___ Remount after processing
___ Repair
___ Reline; rebase [heat cure / self cure]
___ Resilient liner
___ Other ________

Minor connectors		Rests		Clasps			
Tooth no.	Location	Tooth no.	Location	Tooth no.	Type	Location undercut	Amount undercut

OTHER INSTRUCTIONS

____

For dentist's use:
Cost: $

Thank you,
John Doe, D.D.S.

ceptible to the tongue. It also allows the gingival tissues to be free of metal contact. The bar should be approximately 4 to 5 mm wide for adequate rigidity. Therefore, approximately 8 mm of room from the free gingival margin to the floor of the mouth is needed if a lingual bar is to be used. If there is not enough room, a split lingual bar or lingual plating is indicated (Fig. 14-11).

In the maxillary arch, it is important to keep the major connector positioned just behind the most distally prominent rugae whenever possible. The rugae area of the palate is the position where the tongue rests and contacts during most functions (Fig. 14-12). Coverage of this area can lead to patient complaints of bulkiness or speech problems.

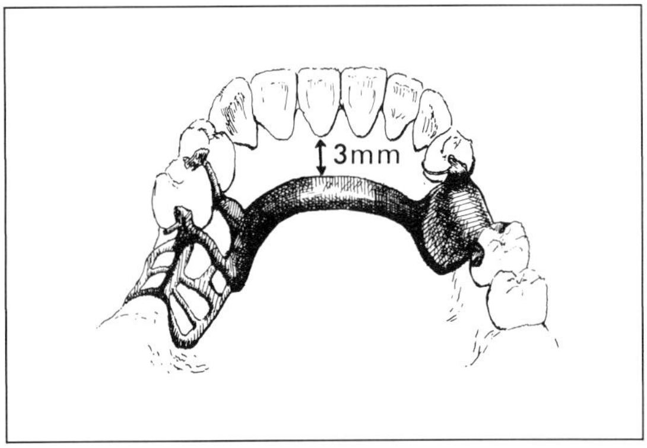

Fig. 14-10 The mandibular lingual bar should be kept at least 3 mm away from the free gingival margin.

Specific designs

Tooth-borne removable partial dentures

Most tooth-borne removable partial dentures can be designed to be comfortable, esthetic, and functional for the patient. This type of removable partial denture gains its stability from the multiple tooth contacts. There are no distal extension areas that will move against the soft tissues of the ridges; therefore, rotations about a fulcrum line are not considered important. The distal extension removable partial dentures are more complex to design because one must consider the rotational movements that the partial denture may have in function.

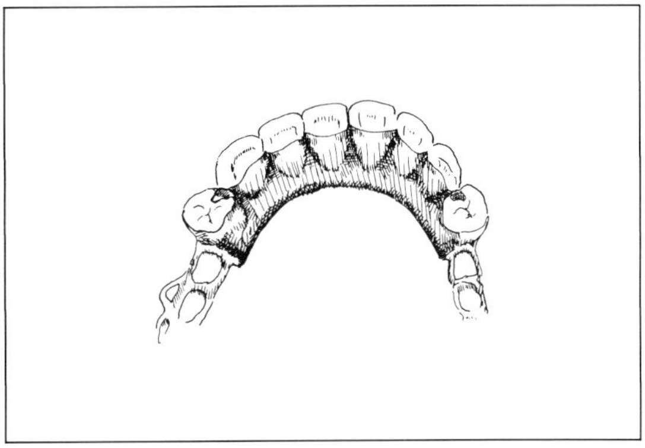

Fig. 14-11 Lingual plating is indicated when there is not enough room for a lingual bar to be used.

Distal extension removable partial dentures

The distal extension of a removable partial denture can move in the mouth in all three dimensions around the vertical, horizontal, or sagittal axes. Vertical or angular forces are applied to the re-

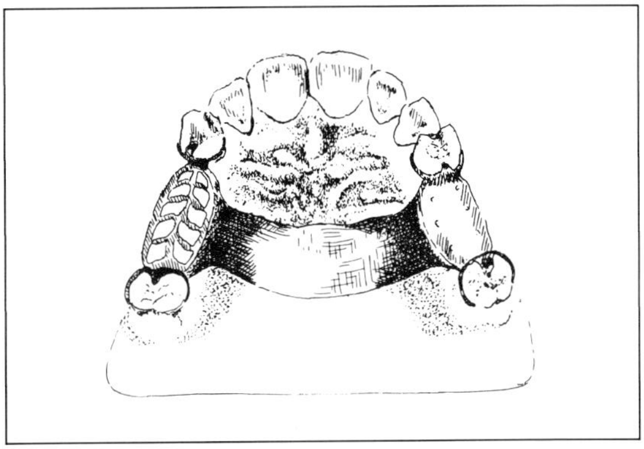

Fig. 14-12 The major connector in the maxilla is kept distal to the most prominent posterior rugae of the palate. This is usually more comfortable for the patient.

Fig. 14-9 *(left)* Dental laboratory work authorization form for removable partial dentures.

movable partial denture during mastication, swallowing, bruxing, or clenching. Unseating forces are directed to the removable partial denture when the stickiness or suction of food lifts the distal extension away from the basal tissue.

When a removable partial denture does not have a distal abutment, we must rely on the residual ridge to provide some of the support for the prosthesis. The remaining teeth do provide some support, but we must keep in mind our primary objective, which is to preserve the remaining structures. To achieve this end we must plan our framework to gain the most benefit from the teeth without overstressing them. We must plan our base coverage to distribute the occlusal load over as wide an area as possible to try to preserve the residual ridge.

Occlusal load upon the removable partial denture is transmitted to the teeth primarily through the rests. As the distal extension denture bases are depressed, the rest can act as the fulcrum for the rotation of the denture (Fig. 14-13). What must be avoided in the design of the removable partial denture is the "seesaw effect" of the rest and clasp assembly. As an occlusal load is placed upon the distal extension area, a Class I lever is put into action (Fig. 14-14). As the denture base is depressed, the clasp can put undue stress on the tooth. A distal extension removable partial denture requires a design that will not put undue stress on the teeth.

One way of helping to distribute the stress is to move the occlusal rest to a tooth anterior to it[2,3] (Fig. 14-15). Then, when the distal extension base is depressed under occlusal load, the denture will rotate on this anterior rest, while the clasp arm will move towards the gingiva into an area of lesser undercut (Fig. 14-16).

This design concept is similar to the RPA clasp design discussed by Eliason.[4] The *R* is the mesial rest, the *P* is the proximal plate, and the A is an Akers or circumferential clasp. The design concept discussed here differs from the RPA design only in the fact that the rest seat is placed more anteriorly.

Regardless of design approach, a conscious effort must be made to appropriately distribute the stresses between the teeth and the edentulous areas.

Use of stone indices to control tooth positions with removable partial dentures

It is not uncommon to find that tooth positions in removable partial dentures are difficult to achieve if the positioning of the teeth is an afterthought—that is, if it occurs after the partial denture framework has been cast. The casting is usually made without considering where the teeth will be positioned on it. The framework metal can interfere with positioning the tooth where it will look best and function properly. Sometimes the retentive areas of the meshwork must be ground to fit the tooth into place, thereby reducing or eliminating the retention mechanism. The teeth may have to be ground excessively to fit them into place. This could easily alter esthetic tooth size or contour. Because of these problems, the denture teeth usually end up being positioned too far to the buccal or facial surfaces. The necks of the teeth are often positioned out at the buccal surface.

Another problem also occurs. Because the dentist and laboratory technician do not know the ultimate precise tooth position, it is common to create an external finishing line that is too far from the teeth. This creates an area of additional bulk of material where it is not needed and where it will make the patient uncomfortable. If the tooth position could be determined prior to the casting of the framework, then it would be possible to locate the finishing line closer to the denture teeth with less bulk.

Determining anterior tooth positions for a removable partial denture must begin during the diagnostic phase. During the patient visit in which diagnostic impressions are made, the mold and shade for the anterior teeth to be replaced should be selected. After the casts are poured, an acrylic resin template is made upon the cast so that denture teeth can be set up and waxed to it for a try-in.

During the subsequent patient visit, the acrylic resin template with the denture teeth attached is tried in the patient's mouth to determine satisfaction with tooth color, form, and position. Instruct the patient to stand in front of a large wall mirror. This is an excellent opportunity to demonstrate to the patient the esthetic result of a removable partial

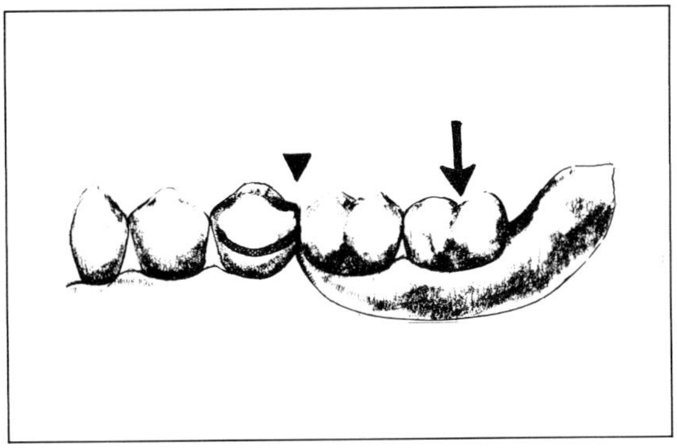

Fig. 14-13 The most distal rest areas in this situation will be the fulcrum about which the removable partial denture will rotate.

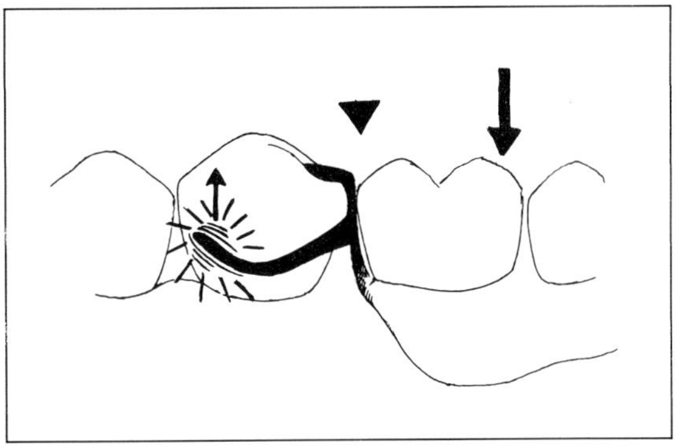

Fig. 14-14 When the distal extension is depressed, a Class I lever is put into action with this clasp/rest combination. This could traumatize the tooth.

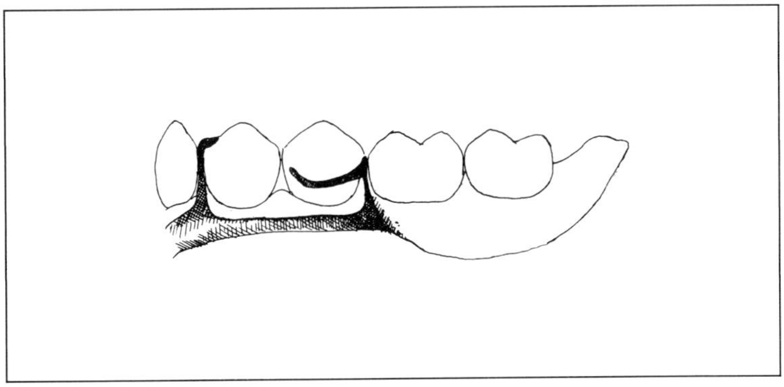

Fig. 14-15 The rest is moved anterior to the most distal abutment. The distal abutment is clasped but not rested upon.

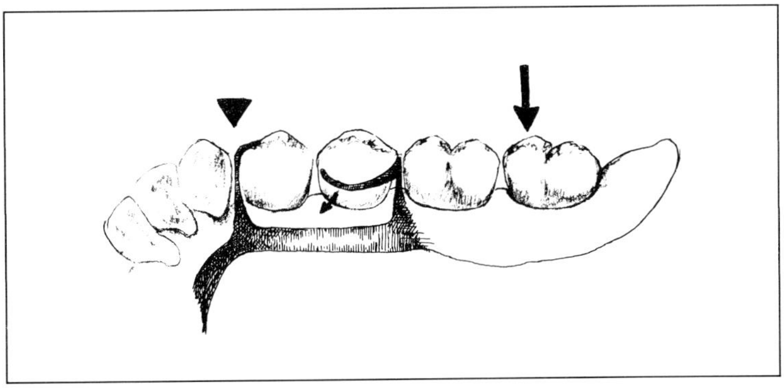

Fig. 14-16 When the distal extension base is depressed, rotation will take place about the anteriorly placed rest. The clasp on the most distal abutment will not torque the tooth because the entire clasp assembly will move toward the gingiva.

denture *prior* to actually making it. This procedure eliminates many insertion-day surprises for the patient and dentist.

The laboratory technician can use this template wax-up as a guide for the tooth positions. A stone index of the tooth positions can be made by lubricating the labial surfaces of the stone anterior teeth and then flowing stone onto the denture teeth and the adjacent stone (natural) teeth. The index is removed when set and trimmed to size. Write the word "index" on it and send it to the laboratory technician. During the wax-up of the removable partial denture upon the refractory (investment) cast, the technician can position the index on it as a guide for finishing the wax-up.

Use of completed bases for removable partial dentures

As with complete dentures, the more accurate the bases are, the more accurate jaw relation records will be. For this reason it is sometimes important to process and complete the denture bases upon the framework prior to making jaw relation records. The laboratory procedures for making the completed bases are quite similar to those procedures outlined in chapter 7 for complete dentures.

The use of a functional impression and an altered cast technique for Kennedy Class I, II, and some IV designs is very important. The functional impression provides for a decrease in mobility to counteract the forces that are applied to the prosthesis. Better adaptation of the denture borders can be attained by border molding. The following is an outline of the steps required to make processed acrylic resin completed bases for removable partial dentures after a functional impression has been made:

1. Bead the final impression of the edentulous areas using beading or utility wax. Baseplate wax can be seated to this wax to fill in the tongue space areas.
2. Fill in the impressioned area with stone. Make a mound of the same mix of stone, and invert the removable partial denture onto it. Adapt the soft stone to the removable partial denture framework to contact as much of its surface as possible without locking it into place. Do not allow any stone to flow into areas that will make separation difficult.
3. Allow the stone to set. Separate the impression from the cast. It is usually necessary to place the stone in a hot-water bath to warm and soften the impression materials used. Remove all traces of the tray acrylic resin and impression materials.
4. Reposition the framework on the cast and secure it in place with sticky wax.
5. Place strips of utility wax in the peripheral border areas to ensure adequate thickness to the border areas and slopes of the ridges. The thickness of the wax will be the ultimate thickness of the acrylic resin when it is later boiled out and flasked with the acrylic resin.
6. Adapt one sheet of baseplate wax over the entire edentulous ridge area and over the utility wax up to the land areas of the cast.
7. Flask and process the acrylic resin in the same manner as you would process acrylic resin bases for complete dentures (chapter 7). Deflask the removable partial denture with the attached completed bases in the conventional manner. Trim and adjust the acrylic resin as needed, and place a butt joint finishing line in the acrylic resin as is done for complete dentures (chapter 7).
8. Prepare the original master cast by cutting off the edentulous stone areas where the acrylic resin processed base was added to the framework. Place retentive grooves in the stone along its edges. Reposition the framework with the attached base back on the master cast, and check for its complete seating. Secure the framework on the cast with sticky wax. Adapt Play-Doh to the inside of the denture base to block out any undercuts.
9. Soak the cast in a supersaturated solution of calcium sulfate for 15 minutes. Pour fast-setting stone into the processed base to form a mounting cast for this area as is done for complete dentures (chapter 7). The result is an altered cast.
10. Evaluate the fit of the attached completed bases in the patient's mouth prior to making any jaw relation records. Pressure-indicating paste can be used to determine any pressure areas or border

overextensions. Establish the maxillomandibular jaw relation records, and arrange and try in the teeth as you would complete dentures. Complete the final wax-up around the teeth and up to the butt joint of the completed base. Perform the second processing of the removable partial denture in the same manner as for complete dentures (chapter 12).

Use of checkpoints with removable partial dentures

The Centric Check Points described for use with complete dentures (chapter 8) are also useful for verification of centric jaw relation with removable partial dentures. When a centric checkpoint cannot oppose a checkpoint in the opposing arch, the point can be set up to touch a cusp tip or another easily identifiable point on the tooth. A centric checkpoint can also be attached to a distal extension processed base to touch a centric checkpoint in the opposing arch. In each of these instances, no cups are used to set the checkpoints. They are positioned manually to touch the selected points.

References

1. Jermyn, A.C. Machine-controlled tooth preparation for inlays and bridgework. Dent. Digest 68:454–459, 1962.
2. Steffel, V.L. Fundamental principles involved in partial denture design. J. Am. Dent. Assoc. 42:534–544, 1951.
3. Avant, E.W. Indirect retention in partial denture design. J. Prosthet. Dent. 16:1103–1110, 1966.
4. Eliason, C.M. RPA clasp design for distal-extension removable partial dentures. J. Prosthet. Dent. 49:25, 1983.

I ran a survey of 1,000 patients that presented for a removable partial denture adjustment. Of these patients, the vast majority had the same problem—they could not get their own natural teeth to contact. A rest, a clasp, or a tooth on the removable partial denture kept the patient from bringing his own teeth together. The occlusion was not carefully checked after the insertion of the prosthesis.

Allen Brewer
(Personal communication)

Index